A WORK IN PROGRESS

**Behavior Management Strategies and a Curriculum
for Intensive Behavioral Treatment of Autism**

Ron Leaf

John McEachin

A Work in Progress
Copyright © 1999 Autism Partnership

Published by: DRL Books Inc.
                 37 East 18th Street, 10th Floor
                 New York, NY 10003
                 Phone: 212 604 9637
                 Fax: 212 206 9329

Book Design: John Eng
Editorial Technician: Sue Lee
Cover Art: Ramon Gil

Copyright 1999 by Ron Leaf and John McEachin

Library of Congress Control Number: 2008902086
ISBN: 978-0-9665266-0-8

Printed in the United States of America

Table of Contents

Behavioral Strategies For Teaching And Improving Behavior Of Autistic Children

---

The Autism Partnership Curriculum for Discrete Trial Teaching with Autistic Children

■ Appendices

Preface

This book has been more than 20 years in the making and it is still not finished. We consider it a work in progress. Even as these words are being written, one of our talented staff or a dedicated parent is out there somewhere thinking of a new and clever way to teach an important skill to an autistic child. But if we waited until we thought we had included all the useful programs, this book would never be published.

What we have tried to do is provide a road map and enough detailed examples that people working with autistic children might develop a good understanding of the teaching process. This is not a cookbook and should not be treated as such. Every autistic child is different and the program needs to be tailored accordingly. Not every program need be done with every child. Some children will need many additional programs beyond what is included in this book. One must proceed with flexibility and learn from the child. We want people to feel comfortable developing and trying out new teaching programs. As long as you are guided by the data, you will not go far astray. That is the beauty of Applied Behavior Analysis.

Although still far from complete, the body of knowledge about effective intervention and teaching techniques that has been assembled by dedicated researchers is truly impressive. We have built upon the work of other people, just as we expect that people will build upon the work we present here. We have benefitted from the insights and innovations of the most talented teachers in the world. Some of them are certified professionals, including special education teachers and speech pathologists. Many of them are paraprofessionals. Still others are parents who have a gift for understanding how to reach their children.

We have been heavily influenced by the work of Ivar Lovaas at UCLA, where we spent many years learning under his mentoring. He has written a classic work that everyone in this field should know about, *Teaching Developmentally Disabled Children: The Me Book*. It's scope is somewhat limited, but the depth of discussion is enlightening even two decades later. A more recent work that has a broad scope is *Behavioral Intervention For Young Children With Autism*, edited by Catherine Maurice. For children at advanced stages of the program, *Teach Me Language* by Sabrina

Freeman is indispensable. We hope that our work in progress will earn a place on bookshelves next to those important works.

Ron Leaf   Seal Beach, California

John McEachin   January, 1999

Behavioral Strategies for Teaching and Improving Behavior of Autistic Children

Ron Leaf

John McEachin

Jamison Dayharsh

Marlene Boehm

Partnership

"Autism Partnership" was the name we chose for our agency because of our conviction that working collaboratively with all those involved in the treatment of an individual is vital to success. This does not mean everyone needs to be in constant agreement. A variety of perspectives can be beneficial to the treatment process. Many times there is more than one route that can be followed to the same destination. Constructive debate can bring enlightenment.

Parents, probably more than anyone, can attest to how destructive it is to a child's welfare when there is not collaboration. As professionals we cannot ever really know how frustrating and upsetting conflicts are when one's own child is at the center of the disagreement. For many parents, this is just one more piece of a bad dream that they have been experiencing for years.

One Parent's Story

The nightmare started with the nagging realization that something was not right with the way our son was developing. This must be every parent's greatest fear. We tried to reassure ourselves with the positive indications that everything was fine. Our son had no physical evidence of problems and he had successfully passed most of the early developmental milestones. We kept hearing, "So he's not talking yet . . . . Children talk at different times." Perhaps it was because this is our youngest child. He was not as social as others, but every child is different, with distinct personalities and temperaments. We wanted to downplay the suspicions. We needed to. We had to. Family members and friends were always eager to help deny the fears. But the nagging feeling just did not go away.

We shared our concern with the pediatrician—someone we trusted and who had aided in our children's care and well being. He said not to worry. All children develop a little differently. That was the reassurance we were hoping for and we so wanted to believe it. "Maybe I'm just being an anxious parent and that may be contributing to the problem," I would say to myself. Maybe I'm doing too much for this child—he is the youngest and they say that can happen with the baby of the family.

But in the passing months, things did not improve. The gap between our boy and our friends' children continued to widen. At the next checkup I again reported the lack of progress. One more time I was told not to worry. There would still be plenty of time for him to talk. The doctor smiled reassuringly and said once he starts talking, we would probably wish he would be quiet.

One final time my husband and I went together. We pleaded our case with the pediatrician. Maybe it was just to placate us, but he made a referral. I did not know what to feel. *Comfort?* Someone finally agreed with us and now something finally can happen. *Anger?* I have known something was wrong and no one would listen. *Denial?* Perhaps the pediatrician is now overreacting and everything is actually OK. *Guilt?* Why did I not follow my gut instincts sooner?

What I felt was panic, wanting to get help for our son immediately. Scheduling to see professionals, however, proved trying with long waits for appointments and delays that I was beginning to realize he could ill afford. The first professional we met with very coolly and quickly told us that it was autism. I was devastated, not fully understanding what it meant and all the ramifications, but I knew it was not good. I had actually suspected something like this, but to have the diagnosis was shattering.

I know some parents are not even as "fortunate" as us to get the diagnosis at such an early age. They are told their child is too young, there is nothing out of the ordinary, the doctor does not see any problem, or at least there is nothing outside of the norm that their child will not outgrow. Without a definitive diagnosis they have bounced from diagnostician to diagnostician, being provided with alternative and sometimes competing or contradictory explanations for what is occurring with their child. Some parents are given an incorrect diagnosis that sends them down the wrong path altogether.

Having such experiences in dealing with professionals, all we can think about is the precious time that our child has lost. You are already feeling tormented and then along come well-meaning family and friends that question the diagnosis. You are so tempted to join them in their disbelief, but deep in your heart you know the best thing to do is not listen to them. Their well-meaning skepticism does not help ease the pain. You do not have the time or energy to debate and try to convince them.

The nightmare continued. We suffered the pain of not receiving invitations to join in-group activities because unspoken concerns about how our boy would behave. Our circle of friends diminished as we spent increasing time seeking information and treatment. Social activities were difficult to enjoy anyway and the birthday party of another child was only a painful reminder of the deficits in our own child. Friends could not have known what to say and their encouragement would sound shallow. I felt isolated, helpless, and lost.

Finally, there came an overwhelming need to regroup. Gathering all my strength, I started trying to sort out the options. Where do you even start looking for helpful information about autism? The little I found sounded bleak. There were tremendous contradictions and what later turned out to be misinformation. I read that it is a life long disorder and that our child would always be seriously impaired. Then there were all the supposed "cures." Who was I to believe? You want to believe that recovery is an option, but you fear it is not really possible. The nightmare continued.

There are such strong and diverse opinions. Vitamin therapies, diets, allergy treatments, play therapy, sensory integration, TEACCH or Lovaas? There are even some interventions that seem so outrageous they gave me a good laugh. And then there are all the therapies: speech, occupational, play, physical and behavioral. You are told with such conviction that one is absolutely the best and the others may be quite harmful. Then you get a second opinion, which of course is exactly the opposite. You want to scream!

It seemed that there was little that would be truly effective and we would just have to accept the diagnosis and bleak prognosis. We choose special education, hoping that our child could at least learn something and be happy. A year later I read something about behavioral treatment and for some reason this time it made me really think. When I questioned the professionals, they said no, it's just not the miracle we were looking for, that we were already doing everything that could help him. But when I talked to a few parents who were actually doing an intensive behavioral program it seemed like there must be something to this. Their children had made amazing progress. When I did more research on my own I found books and scientific articles that provide convincing proof that these anti-behavioral professionals once again were incorrect. The nightmare was ending, but a long road of hard work lay ahead of us.

Once a parent decides upon a treatment, all too often the nightmare intensifies. The absence of partnership becomes blatantly apparent. Who is responsible for providing what? Which treatment should take a higher priority? How many hours of intervention does my child need? Once again, parents are put in the center of disagreement. Not only is this a continuation of the emotional turmoil they have been experiencing for years, but it can also sabotage effective treatment.

There are a number of agencies that provide quality treatment for individuals with autism. However, even among those that have vast Applied Behavior Analysis (ABA) experience, there are usually variations. Differences in treatment practices are a likely function of multiple factors such as the ages of the children served, treatment settings, functioning level of clients as well as individual philosophies and varying interpretation of research. Professionals from different disciplines are likely to make conflicting recommendations, particularly if they are not familiar with the most current research on ABA. This can be especially confusing for parents who have to decide on a treatment approach for their child. For those who have chosen to implement an ABA program, they will fortunately find that there is far more agreement than disagreement among ABA providers. The choice of a specific ABA clinic may come down to choosing the agency whose philosophy makes you feel most comfortable. Because of the experiences that parents all too often have to suffer through, it is not surprising that they are skeptical at best, and more likely suspicious, distrusting and furious toward professionals. It is a natural reaction to an intolerable situation. And then professionals are surprised and do not understand why parents are so angry and distrusting!

We must work together. We have to agree to disagree. We have to rely upon data that supports treatment effectiveness. We have to focus on the child. We have to value the unique blend that comes from incorporating all the perspectives within a team. We have to work as a partnership.

Intensive Behavioral Intervention

Autism is a severe disruption of the normal developmental processes that occurs in the first two years of life. It leads to impaired language, play, cognitive, social and adaptive functioning, causing children to fall farther and farther behind their peers as they grow older. The cause is unknown, but evidence points to physiological causes such as neurological abnormalities to certain areas of the brain.

Autistic children do not learn in the same way that other children normally learn. They seem unable to understand simple verbal and nonverbal communication, are confused by sensory input, and withdraw in varying degrees from people and the world around them. They become preoccupied with certain activities and objects that interfere with development of play. They show little interest in other children and tend not to learn by observing and imitating others.

Despite the disruption of learning processes, behavioral scientists, relying on the principles of learning theory, have developed effective methods for teaching autistic children. Three decades of research by Dr. Ivar Lovaas and his associates at UCLA have convincingly demonstrated that intensive, early intervention can significantly improve the functioning of autistic children. Two follow-up studies, published in 1987 and 1993, have shown that 9 of the 19 children who received intensive behavioral treatment were able to successfully complete regular education classes and were indistinguishable from their peers on measures of IQ, adaptive skills, and emotional functioning. Even among those children who did not attain the best outcome, there were significant gains in language, social, self-help and play skills, and all but two of the children developed functional speech.

The children in this study were up to three years old when treatment started. They received an **AVERAGE** of 40 man-hours per week of individual treatment provided by UCLA undergraduates who were supervised by graduate students and psychologists. Treatment lasted an average of two years or longer.

HISTORICAL FOUNDATIONS

Applied Behavior Analysis (ABA) with autistic children has experienced a return to popularity since 1993. This popularity, in large part, can be linked to the publication of Catherine Maurice's book, *Let Me Hear Your Voice*, in which she chronicles the treatment of her two autistic children. Like many professionals and parents, Ms. Maurice initially had a dim view of behavioral intervention. She believed it to be an extremely negative and inflexible procedure. Moreover, she thought that behavioral intervention had limited effectiveness and often produced children with a robotic manner. Her experience, however, proved to be far different. She found that behavioral intervention can be employed positively with a high degree of flexibility. Most important, the intervention proved to be tremendously effective.

Ms. Maurice's story gave hope to parents who had been led to believe, often by professionals, that autistic children will always remain severely impacted by their disorder. With hope and a direction, parents throughout the world started setting up intensive behavioral programs. Parents also started demanding that schools and state agencies use ABA with their children.

Although the tremendous popularity of ABA is recent, ABA is not a new procedure. Critics of behavioral intervention often contend that it is an "experimental" procedure with limited empirical evidence of its effectiveness. Lovaas (1987) and McEachin, Smith and Lovaas (1993) are cited as the only two investigations that show the effectiveness of behavioral intervention with autistic children. In fact, ABA is based upon more than 50 years of scientific investigation with individuals affected by a wide range of behavioral and developmental disorders. Since the early '60s, extensive research has proved the efficacy of behavioral intervention with autistic children, adolescents and adults. The research has shown ABA to be effective in reducing disruptive behaviors typically observed in autistic individuals, such as self-injury, tantrums, noncompliance and self-stimulation. ABA has also been shown to be effective in teaching commonly deficient skills such as complex communication, social, play and self-help skills. Lovaas and his colleagues (1973) published a comprehensive study that demonstrated ABA to be effective in treating multiple behaviors with multiple children.

Although the work by Lovaas is the most frequently cited, there is other evidence that ABA can result in substantial benefit. Harris and Handleman (1994) reviewed several research studies that showed that more than 50% of autistic children who participated in comprehensive preschool programs using ABA were successfully integrated into non-handicapped classrooms, with many requiring little ongoing treatment.

CURRICULUM

The objective of intervention is to teach your child those skills that will facilitate his development and help him achieve the greatest degree of independence and the highest quality of life possible. Several curricula exist that delineate a variety of skills. Curricula have been developed through decades of research.

The content of the curriculum should include all the skills a person needs to be able to function successfully and to enjoy life to its fullest. It should include teaching skills that most children typically do not need to be formally taught such as play and imitation. A strong emphasis should be placed on learning to talk, the development of conceptual and academic skills, and promoting play and social skills. However, as a child gets older, the emphasis should shift to practical knowledge and adaptive skills. The curriculum should be developmentally sequenced so that easier concepts and skills are taught first and complex skills are not introduced until the child has learned the prerequisite skills. However, there should not be rigid adherence to a preconceived notion of the order in which children should learn. For example, although it is not the usual pattern, some children learn to read before they can talk.

It is important to build on a child's successes and expand the utilization of existing skills as well as encourage the development of new ones. Development of verbal communication will not relieve the child's needs in the areas of play, social skills and adaptive functioning. Instruction designed specifically to teach these areas is essential! Some children may never learn to talk and will need some alternate means of communication. The overall approach is empirical and pragmatic: if it works, stick with it; if it does not work, change it.

HOW MANY HOURS OF INTERVENTION SHOULD MY CHILD RECEIVE?

In deciding how many hours of therapy to schedule per week, you should look at your child's day and attempt to provide a reasonable balance between intensive therapy, periods of less intensive activities that are still structured, and allowance for your child's need to have periods of free time and family time. Besides the number of hours of one-to-one teaching, you should consider the quality of teaching and the degree of structure provided outside the formal therapy hours. Research shows that many children will do best with 30 or more hours per week of direct instruction. The length of therapy sessions should be adjusted to provide maximum benefit. Often it will work best to keep it in the range of two to three hours.

The introduction of play dates will be necessary to generalize skills and provide observational learning opportunities. Once your child is spending part of the day in school, it may be advisable to reduce the therapy hours at home.

WHAT IS THE FAMILY'S ROLE?

The involvement of the family is critical in the treatment process. No one knows your child better than you and you are ultimately the ones who care the most and are most affected by your child's disorder. You spend a great deal of time with your child and you can use that time to generalize the teaching goals into everyday living situations.

Parents often provide direct therapy to their child. However, as parents know all too well, living with an autistic child takes a big emotional toll and coordinating the treatment team is a big job. Therefore, whenever possible, it is recommended to use hired therapists to do most of the intensive work. This allows parents to have some respite and the remaining time spent with their child can be more enjoyable and productive. Parents can use the child's time that is not spent in intensive programming to develop play, social and self-help skills. Outings to the park, grocery shopping, mailing a letter and visits to a relative's home are opportunities to generalize skills and work on improving behavior. Similarly, bath time, dinner, getting dressed, and feeding the cat are just a few examples of everyday routines that serve as opportunities for teaching. In this way, the child's entire day becomes part of the therapy process and the parents become an integral part of the team. It is important to involve the child in the daily routine of living, therefore pushing against further isolation.

THERAPY FORMAT

Teaching is a process that will change over time. Initially, the duration of time spent in formal discrete trial teaching will steadily increase as your child becomes comfortable with intervention. In later stages, the amount of time spent in discrete trials will decrease as time in other types of instruction increases (e.g., group and incidental teaching). Curriculum emphasis will also shift during the course of therapy. However, therapy's general structure will remain the same. Intervention will be a combination of programs designed to increase communication, play, social, and self-help skills. Every child's program should be individualized to his or her particular needs. However, the following is an example of how time might be allocated in a typical three-hour therapy shift:

20 minutes	Structured Play (inside)
80 minutes	Language (short breaks throughout: 0-20 minutes language; 5-10 minutes play; 0-20 minutes language; 5-10 minutes play; etc.)
30 minutes	Self-Help Skills
30 minutes	Structured Play (outside)
20 minutes	Record Completion and Debriefing

Any part of this distribution may be increased or decreased depending upon the child's age, the stage of therapy, and school requirements.

TEACHING FORMAT

Applied Behavior Analysis should be the major treatment modality employed in the program. Although many different techniques may be used as part of treatment, the primary instructional method should be *Discrete Trial Teaching* (DTT). This is a specific methodology used to maximize learning. It is a teaching process that can be used to develop most skills, including cognitive, communication, play, social and self-help skills. Additionally, it is a strategy that can be used for all ages and populations.

DISCRETE TRIAL TEACHING IS NOT A TEACHING STRATEGY THAT IS USED ONLY FOR TEACHING LANGUAGE, NOR IS IT ONLY EMPLOYED FOR YOUNG CHILDREN WITH AUTISM.

IT IS SIMPLY GOOD TEACHING!!!

DTT involves: 1) breaking a skill into smaller parts; 2) teaching one sub-skill at a time until mastery; 3) allowing repeated practice in a concentrated period of time; 4) providing prompting and prompt fading as necessary; and 5) using reinforcement procedures.

The basic teaching unit, called a *trial*, has a distinct beginning and end, hence the name "discrete." Teaching involves numerous trials in order to strengthen learning. Each part of the skill is mastered before more information is presented. In discrete trial teaching, a very small unit of information is presented and the student's response is immediately sought. The student must be active and engaged during learning. This contrasts with continuous trial or more traditional teaching methods which present large amounts of information with no clearly defined target response on the student's part.

Other techniques used in treatment may include behavior management, crisis intervention, structured teaching interactions, and more traditional counseling methods.

TEACHING SETTINGS

Initially, teaching is done in an environment that will lead to early success. Sometimes that may mean removing distractions. However, teaching must quickly be extended to ordinary environments. Not only is this more natural but it also promotes transferring learning to all settings. Therefore, therapy should occur THROUGHOUT the entire house as well as outside and in the community at such places as the park, McDonald's, and the market. If distractions pose a problem, it will be critical that your child be taught to focus despite environmental interference. Children must be able to learn in varied environments where distractions naturally occur so as to prepare them for learning in typical settings such as school.

STAGES OF THERAPY

As your child learns, therapy will progress through different stages. Although the stages are not absolutely distinct, therapy can be described in three phases:

Beginning Stages involve getting to know your child. It is critical to establish a warm, playful and reinforcing social relationship. To help accomplish this goal, the first month of therapy emphasizes identification and establishment of reinforcers, with much play and noncontingent delivery of reinforcers. Through creating a positive atmosphere, your child will be far more amenable to the teaching process and therefore proceed faster through therapy with fewer power struggles and disruptive behaviors. It is essential to determine your child's likes and dislikes as well as identifying his strengths and weaknesses. **"Learning to Learn"** is also a critical component of the beginning stage. The child needs to learn that cooperation with requests will result in immediate and frequent rewards. This further entails acquiring skills such as learning how to sit and attend, remaining on task in the teaching situation, being responsive to instruction, learning how to process feedback, and understanding cause and effect. This sets the stage for learning concepts and skills.

Middle Stages of therapy involve learning specific communication, play, self-help and social skills. Complex concepts are broken down into a series of steps that are taught systematically. Abstract concepts are translated into concrete examples. As the child moves through the program, there will be individualized adjustment of the curriculum to meet your child's needs. Although the initial goal is to rapidly accelerate skill development, the long-term goal is to increase the child's ability to learn and function in natural settings. Therefore, therapy should be done as naturally as possible in order to promote the long term goal without comprising the child's learning rate. Children should be exposed to play dates and other social and community settings. Children are usually introduced to the school setting during this stage.

Advanced Stages involve progressively making therapy more natural and generalizable to the everyday environment. Working on subtler social, play, affective, cognitive and communication skills is the primary focus during this stage. Completion of integration into natural learning environments (i.e., school) also occurs at this time.

EVALUATION

The effectiveness of therapy must be continually evaluated. Staff should collect data daily. Information should be specific to both teaching programs and behaviors. Regular team meetings are the forums for reviewing the effectiveness of intervention and making program refinements. Video taping at home at least once a month is highly recommended.

PROGRAM EFFECTIVENESS

Intervention has been shown to successfully increase children's functioning in areas such as language, play, social and self-help. Naturally, however, there is a range in the degree of treatment outcomes. The result of treatment depends upon several factors including age at onset of treatment, quality of treatment, the child's cognitive capacity and consistency in the home environment. Treatment is designed to bring out the child's fullest potential.

Although "recovery" is naturally the desired outcome, research findings suggest that less than half of children who begin treatment before age three can achieve such a result under optimal conditions. However, nearly all the children studied made substantial progress including development of communication, social and play skills. It is difficult to determine in advance which children will respond most favorably to treatment. Presence of communication skills and overall degree of cognitive ability prior to treatment are correlated with outcome. However, the rate of learning once treatment commences is a more reliable predictor and after six months of treatment, you will have an idea of how quickly the child will progress in treatment.

FACTORS THAT GOOD PROGRAMS HAVE IN COMMON

1. Consistency inside and outside of therapy

2. Minimum of two hours a week of supervision

3. Parents and staff attend all meetings

4. Training of new staff occurs prior to treatment

5. Parental appreciation of therapy team

6. Pleasant working environment

7. Problems are discussed with the Supervisor

8. Not comparing children

9. Not comparing staff

10. Appreciating different therapists' styles

11. Flexibility in scheduling

12. Parental participation in a portion of therapy sessions

13. Open communication among all members of the team

14. Active, creative question asking and problem solving

A Method That Works For Older Children And Adolescents Too

While it may be true that the best time to start treatment is at a very young age, most older children also can benefit from intensive treatment. Working with older children, however, necessitates building on previous efforts by adapting and refining the treatment model. Adjustments are not only necessary in an older child's treatment but also in communicating with his parents.

Parents of older autistic children have often had fundamentally different experiences than parents of younger children. They have had to endure for a much longer time the tremendous challenges of parenting a severely disabled child. For years they have been trying to work through the maze of treatment options, treatment fads and professional feuding. They may have had to endure prolonged frustration over not receiving adequate services. Often they experience intense feelings of helplessness, hopelessness, and anger at seeing their child age with little improvement. Successful intervention with families of older children will need to address parents' concerns, frustrations and anger. It also should combine intensive intervention with parental counseling and education to address and resolve these long festering issues.

First and foremost, it is essential to listen to and attempt to understand the parents' struggles as well as guide them on how to work more successfully with the system. This often requires providing parents information, identifying resources, or helping them establish support systems. Sorting out their experiences is also important. Parents of older children have often been inundated with inaccurate information. It is essential therefore, to provide accurate information and clarify their perceptions. This often means addressing their understanding of diagnosis, etiology, treatment and prognosis. It is rare that a parent has not been caught up in some purported "cure of the year." This often means dealing with a parent's grieving and anger over having an autistic child.

Perhaps the most important aspect of working with parents is dealing with their expectations regarding their child's prognosis. Parents need guidance in formulating realistic expectations. Some parents greatly overestimate their child's potential and maintain a high level of denial. Others are far too pessimistic and have bought into the prevailing wisdom that there is little one can do to improve the fate of an autistic child. Although prognosis carries a high level of uncertainty, they should maintain a level of optimism tempered with realism. Although this also applies to parents of younger children, it is especially important for parents of older children for whom the uncertainties of adulthood loom closer.

Helping parents deal with their child's behaviors and skill deficits is an important element in the treatment of older children. Older children often present a higher frequency and intensity of disruptive behaviors, which is more difficult to manage. We have found it important to train parents in the application of behavior management techniques outside of intensive direct instruction for the child. Whereas the bulk of treating younger children occurs in one-on-one structured therapy, treatment of older children entails a greater need for parents to provide intervention in the context of less formal interaction throughout the child's day. We have de-emphasized the parents' role in providing discrete trial teaching in order to concentrate their efforts on "therapy outside of therapy." For example, dealing with their child's acting out behavior in the community or facilitating his language while in the car, or assisting in his play at the park is every bit as important as the work in formal discrete trial sessions.

Working with older children requires having an eye toward practicality. It means helping parents *fit therapy into their life, not their life into therapy*. It requires assessing the family's needs and helping them set priorities. It is essential not to increase their burdens but to recognize and understand their particular situation and therefore provide therapy in the context of their family's needs. It often requires identifying practical alternatives, problem solving and helping them understand how to teach within their primary role as parents. It still means designing a treatment program that does not compromise effectiveness but also must not add to the family's already challenging and difficult situation. Therefore, identification and utilization of all resources including recruiting and training paraprofessionals has been an essential component in the treatment of older children and adolescents.

WORKING WITH OLDER CHILDREN

Problems Associated with Older Children
- Behavior Problems And Physical Size
- Longer Time For Behaviors To Become Ingrained
- May Need To Address Priority Behaviors
- Splintering Of Skills (e.g., reads but does not dress self)
- Reinforcement Issues (e.g., age-appropriateness)

Need to be Flexible and Creative
- Greater Reliance On School As Setting For Program
- Utilize Available Resources
- Revealing Diagnosis **MAY** Elicit Greater Cooperation From Service Providers
- Guidelines For Teaching (e.g., should trials be less discrete?)
- Structure Of Therapy (e.g., two hours per day of DTT?)

Curriculum Issues
- Greater Emphasis On Recreational And Social Skills
- Functional (Non-speech) Communication If Needed
- Self-help And Daily Living Skills
- Community Access

Accommodate the Need for Increased Independent Functioning
- Indirect Cuing For Attending Behavior
- Make As Naturalistic As Possible
- Avoid Dependence On One-to-One Aide
- Do Not Focus Only On Discrete Trial Discrimination Training/Academics
- Teach Functional Skills
- Big Emphasis On Play And Social

Specialized Therapies
- Counseling
- Systematic Desensitization
- Social Skills Training

✐ Multidisciplinary Approach (O.T./Speech/Etc.)
✐ Sexuality Training

Role of Parents
✐ Oversee/Coordinate Team
✐ Generalize: Supermarket, Bath time, Incidental teaching (play, social)
✐ Not To Feel Guilty Over Missed Opportunities

Realistic Expectations
✐ Aim For Maximizing Potential

EDUCATIONAL PLACEMENT

It is the philosophy of Autism Partnership that educational placement should be provided in the least restrictive setting that will enable the child to make the greatest long-term gains. There is a continuum of educational placements available, and therefore it is essential to carefully evaluate which placement best serves the needs of the child. There are advantages and disadvantages with each potential setting and a number of factors are critical in making a determination. It is not necessary to automatically begin in a restrictive placement. Similarly, the team should not automatically rule out a non-inclusive placement. There are times when a more restrictive setting will best meet the child's needs and will enable him to eventually attain a higher level of independence.

The team should consider what is projected to provide the best opportunity to rapidly advance skills in as many domains as possible. Once in a placement, there needs to be continuous evaluation to determine the earliest opportunity to advance to a new placement, when that would be of benefit to the child. It is not necessary that a child move only one level at a time. For example, with outstanding progress and the right circumstances, a child could move directly from a self-contained classroom placement to full inclusion. It is also important not to automatically wait until the child has completely settled into a particular setting before considering advancement. Sometimes the additional challenge, more stimulating environment, or increased availability of meaningful reinforcers will enable a child to immediately be more successful in the more advanced setting, even when his adjustment has not been completely satisfactory in the current setting.

CLASSROOM CONTINUUM

MORE RESTRICTIVE						LESS RESTRICTIVE
RESIDENTIAL SCHOOL	HOME BOUND	SELF CONTAINED	REVERSE MAINSTREAMING	MAIN-STREAMING	FULL INCLUSION WITH SUPPORT	NO SUPPORT NEEDED

Reinforcement

Initially, the effectiveness of the program will be largely dependent upon the strength of the reinforcers available for your child. Over time, we will work toward your child not needing artificial reinforcers and natural contingencies. Initially, your child will most likely not find being calm, cooperative or compliant as inherently motivating. Similarly, your child probably will not find speaking, playing or socializing to be internally rewarding either. If he did, he most likely would not have a diagnosable disorder. By initially providing artificial, external reinforcers, we will be better able to develop appropriate behavior.

OBJECTIONS TO REINFORCEMENT

Some people object to the use of reinforcers for various reasons. They may feel that the use of rewards is not natural. This may be because they have witnessed reinforcement being used poorly and without a plan to fade their use. All people are motivated by reinforcement. Be it a paycheck, vacations, hobbies, or the company of others, we are fulfilled because of the reinforcers that operate in our lives.

There is often opposition to using rewards because of the belief that it constitutes bribery. However, when one uses reinforcement correctly it is not bribery. In everyday life, bribery would be an inducement to do something improper (as in bribing a public official). In behavioral programming, bribery would be waiting until a person refuses to do something and then negotiate a reward. Another example would be when a child is disruptive and you tell him that if he stops, he will receive a reward. This is not the correct way to use reinforcement. You do not want to remind a person of contingencies during the exhibition of the disruptive behavior. Discussion about reinforcers is in itself rewarding and even this mild form of reinforcement should not occur during disruptive behavior. Announcing the contingency also gives him or her an opportunity to negotiate or consider whether it is worth it for him to exhibit the appropriate behavior. Another kind of situation that can be construed as bribery is the automatic promising of a reward at the time a request is made. This can lead to the person becoming dependent upon the promise of a reward and then declining to perform a requested behavior at any time a reward is **NOT** promised. Even worse is teasing a person with a desired reinforcer but withholding it until the requested behavior occurs. All of these are different from an appropriately negotiated behavioral contract or other appropriate uses of positive reinforcement. Perhaps the most common example of contingent reward in everyday life is the common paycheck. We have yet to hear a person object that his or her weekly or monthly paycheck is a form of bribery.

Objections to the use of reinforcement are also raised based on the belief that the child will become dependent upon rewards. This only occurs when the reinforcers are not faded properly and when natural motivators are not built into the plan. Ideally, a program starts with frequent reinforcement and then quickly fades to natural frequencies of reinforcement.

Another excuse for not using reinforcement with a certain child is the experience that nothing seems to be motivating to him. Often, this occurs when the child receives reinforcers in situations where he does not have to earn them or without regard to his behavior. Eating snacks, watching television, going on outings may be freely available as part of the routine and indeed would not work as a reinforcer under such circumstances. If it is actually the case that there are no effective reinforcers for a child, then the goal must be to establish them. Identifying and developing reinforcers takes time. Even if your child has a variety of reinforcers, it is always worthwhile to cultivate more.

"If you do not have good reinforcers and are not working to establish them, you might as well just go home."

IDENTIFYING AND DEVELOPING REINFORCERS

Simply observing your child may help identify reinforcers. A reinforcer does not have to be elaborate. Often, we are under the false assumption that a reinforcer has to be intricate. Some very small and ordinary things can be made into reinforcers with good "packaging" or a good job of "selling" them with your own enthusiastic response to them. High frequency behaviors, such as listening to music or watching television would constitute likely reinforcers. Anything a person would select in a free choice situation will probably work as a reinforcer. Everyday events such as spending individual time with a parent, going for a walk, or having his or her back rubbed can all be effective motivators.

The first step in developing reinforcers is to simply expose your child to potential reinforcers. Sometimes a child does not know how to operate a toy and therefore does not know how exciting it can be. Often, children do not know that they would actually like a toy, activity or food. Adults certainly can relate to this phenomenon. The thought of a certain food may be disgusting to you, but when you finally have enough nerve to try it, you may discover a new delicacy.

Giving free access to potential reinforcers can also create new reinforcers. Once a person has free access, it may become something the person would be interested in earning more of. Cable Television companies do this. Periodically, they provide customers the opportunity to receive free movie channels. Their experience has been by exposing and giving free access that a percentage of customers will find it reinforcing enough to purchase the service.

Often reinforcers have lost their reinforcing value because of the effect known as satiation. If an individual has too much exposure to a reinforcer it will eventually lose its value. For example, when a person eats too much of a specific food, no matter how much he or she likes it, that person will eventually tire of that food. To guard against satiation and therefore ensure maintenance of the reinforcement value, it is necessary to sometimes make a reward unavailable. This is often difficult when your child still likes the reinforcer. But unless a highly pre-ferred reinforcer is sometimes withheld, you will preclude the possibility of other less potent reinforcers being effective and eventually the person will burn out on the single reinforcer due to satiation. What should be done is to put the highly preferred item into a rotation with other less potent reinforcers, so that the person is not receiving any one item all that often.

It is also recommended to limit access to strong reinforcers so that they are only available at certain times or for specific behaviors. If a child is having problems paying attention in formal therapy, we may use a certain reinforcer that is highly desired only during that time. Not only will this preserve the reinforcement value, but it will also greatly increase the incentive to pay attention. Often we ask parents to lock up certain reinforcers and make them available only during therapy.

An effective way to develop reinforcers is to associate potential reinforcers with estab-lished reinforcers. Through associations, the potential reinforcers will acquire similar reinforc-ing value. For example, that is why we always pair social reinforcement like praise and touch with established reinforcers like food, toys, and activities. Another example would be plying an unenthusiastic young baseball spectator with hot dogs, peanuts and cotton candy, all spread out across several innings.

CATEGORIZING REINFORCERS

Different reinforcers will have different values. Some are just okay and others are "to die for!" It is critical to have a full range of reinforcers so that you can utilize differential reinforcement. That is, you want to provide extraordinary reinforcement for extraordinary behavior, good reinforcement for good behavior and OK reinforcement for OK behavior. In this way you will not only reinforce better behavior, but you will provide incentives for improved performance.

SELECTING REINFORCEMENT SCHEDULES

Typically, in the beginning of a program, reinforcement is provided on a very frequent basis. **INITIALLY**, your child may require reinforcement every few minutes for the **ABSENCE** of disruptive behavior. More important, the **PRESENCE** of appropriate behavior should result in even stronger reinforcement.

Remember that the goal of reinforcement is that it is to be provided at natural frequencies. Although you may initially use continuous reinforcement, it will be critical to quickly move to more intermittent schedules of reinforcement (e.g., every 15 minutes, 30, 60, etc.). Whatever schedule your child is likely to encounter in the natural environment (e.g., in a classroom) should be the ultimate objective. The ultimate goal is for reinforcement to occur at a natural frequency (e.g., daily or even weekly).

The initial schedule should be based upon the baseline rate of the disruptive behaviors. For example, if your child acts out every 15 minutes, then he should receive feedback and reinforcement before 15 minutes (e.g., 10 minutes). In this way, he will actually receive and experience reinforcement. One reason for failure is having a schedule of reinforcement at intervals that are too long. This would mean that far too often, the disruptive behavior occurs before the interval is over and therefore the child will rarely access the reinforcer. Reinforcement cannot work if he never experiences it. Furthermore, a thin schedule of reinforcement causes motivation to be very low.

When the reinforcement schedule is faded, more powerful reinforcers should be used. If you do not provide stronger reinforcement, it is likely that regression will occur. Additionally, there is no incentive to continue to improve. It is critical to not provide overly powerful reinforcement at first. Otherwise you will get trapped, because you will be unable to provide stronger rewards as you "thin" the schedule.

The following is an example of a reinforcement schedule. The scale increases reinforcement from left to right. The time intervals are relative. The shortest interval may be 30 seconds or it might be 15 minutes. As the value of the reinforcement increases toward the right side of the scale, the length of time necessary to earn the reward becomes progressively longer.

5 MINS	15 MINS	30 MINS	60 MINS	1/2 DAY	DAILY
Raisin	1/2 cup Juice	5 Minutes Toy Play	Song	Video	Outing

RULES OF REINFORCEMENT

Perhaps one of the most researched topics in psychology has been the topic of reinforcement. For more than 100 years, psychologists have examined the principles and practice of using reinforcement. Reinforcement has been demonstrated to be not only very effective but essential in changing behavior. The research has resulted in the formulation of rules on how to most effectively use rewards.

Reinforcement occurs throughout our daily lives. Teachers, parents, employers, and coaches generally use rewards. However, they are often utilized in a non-systematic manner. Most provide them without knowing the intricacies of how to most effectively deliver reinforcement. Unfortunately, the effectiveness of rewards is largely dependent upon following such rules.

The "rules of reinforcement" have been described in many books and manuals. The following are what we consider to be the most important guidelines.

1.   Reinforcers Should Be Reinforcing

We often project that others would desire what we like (e.g., chocolate ice cream, country music, golf, etc.) when actually some may not find them to be reinforcers at all. Obviously, if it is actually not reinforcing, then the desired behavior or skill will not increase or at best it will be learned very slowly. Therefore, it is necessary to determine whether what we think would be a reward is actually reinforcing. We need to continuously assess the situation. Does your child appear excited when receiving it? When given a choice, does your child select it? The ultimate test is whether your child will work to earn the item you are offering as a reinforcer.

It is critical to continually monitor whether an item is reinforcing. Unfortunately the value of reinforcers often changes rapidly. Therefore, we must be flexible enough to change reinforcers based upon current preference.

2.   Reinforcement Should Be Contingent

Reinforcers should only be available when the target behavior occurs. Be careful about letting reinforcers be accessed at times other than when the target behavior occurs. This has the effect of diminishing the power of the reinforcer. Therefore, try to select only reinforcers that can be reserved for contingent rewards. Do not select a reinforcer if it cannot be withheld or if its being withheld will create tremendous problems.

There is one exception to this rule. Occasionally it may be helpful to provide noncontingent access to a reinforcer that a child rarely selects in order to increase his interest in that item.

3.   A Variety Of Reinforcers Should Be Used

By providing a variety of reinforcers, you will reduce the likelihood of your child becoming satiated by the reinforcer. This will keep the reinforcers fresh and more powerful. It also provides you the tools by which to provide differential feedback. Even if your child likes a reinforcer, rotate it in combination with less potent reinforcers. Also, never give more reinforcement than is necessary.

Whenever a child has limited reinforcers, select the most preferred reinforcers to be provided contingently upon the most important behavior.

4.   Social Reinforcers Should Be Paired With Primaries

Even if your child does not like social reinforcers such as smiles and praise, by associating them with primary reinforcers (e.g., food, drink, favorite toy, etc.), they will eventually become reinforcing as well. Development of social rewards allows you to eventually intermix socials and primaries and to ultimately fade tangible reinforcers to a very thin schedule. Moreover, social reinforcers are the principal rewards used in everyday settings.

5.   Continuously Develop And Identify Reinforcers

Every day, go through the house and round up some new objects to try; cruise the aisles at Toys-R-Us; try things that have worked with other children. Even if it seems that your child does not like a toy or activity, do not give up.

Look to your child's self-stimulation to guide you in what types of items or activities he would prefer. Children that engage in visual self-stimulation may enjoy a marble maze or liquid timer. Children whose self-stimulation is auditory might find musical tapes, push-button sound books or musical instruments of interest.   Kinesthetic kids often find massages, trampolines and tickle games fun.

Toys that have a cause and effect component are frequently engaging. Toys that have multiple uses can remain useful as your child progresses. Look for items that offer sensory stimulation (e.g., toys that make noises, move, have lights), exploration opportunities (e.g., "pin art") and a wide range of simple to complex uses.

6.   Use Age Appropriate Reinforcers

This will increase your child's peer acceptance. It will also make it less evident that your child is receiving reinforcement. Additionally, it will help in people treating your child age appropriately. It will also help your child think of himself in a more age appropriate way and can help promote more sophisticated interests. Finally, this helps promote generalization because your child is more likely to encounter these reinforcers in the natural environment.

7.   Unpredictability And Novelty Greatly Enhance Reinforcement

As we know, surprises are usually very enjoyable and highly motivating. By creating a grab bag or mystery box, you may provide the child with new reinforcers simply by changing their presentation. This enthusiasm will become associated with the persons, places, and teaching materials from the therapy sessions.

8.   In The Beginning, Reinforcement Should Occur Immediately

Reinforcement is most effective when it occurs within one-half of a second following the behavior. This provides the strongest association between the behavior and the reinforcer, thereby making it clearer for your child what the desired behavior is. Immediacy is also especially important initially when the child is "learning to learn."

Providing reinforcers rapidly reduces the chance that other behaviors will be inadvert-ently reinforced. For example, if you are reinforcing eye contact and you delay providing the reward, you may actually be reinforcing him to turn away. Also, if you reinforce a child a few minutes after the behavior, it is quite possible that he may have forgotten what he did and therefore does not know which behavior to repeat in the future. However, as treatment progresses, you should deliberately let there be an increase in delay of rein-forcement so that your child becomes accustomed to the less powerful schedules of reinforcement that exist in the natural environment.

9. The Reinforcement Schedule Should Be Followed Consistently

Consistency of receiving the reinforcer makes it much more likely that your child will repeat the behavior at the desired rate. The more predictable the reinforcer, the more likely the target behavior will occur. If positive behavior occurs and does not get re-warded or, even worse, if negative behavior occurs and the child gets rewarded anyway, progress will be drastically reduced. As the scheduled frequency of reinforcement is reduced (see below) it still is important that everyone on the team be consistent in imple-menting the schedule in order to get the best results.

10. Reinforcement Should Be Faded Over Time

The longer an intensive reinforcement schedule is maintained, the more difficult it will be to fade and the behavior is more likely to extinguish when the rewards are re-duced. When you have started fading the schedule, there may be times that it becomes necessary to temporarily increase the frequency or reinforcement if your child is experi-encing problems. Also, as the schedule is thinned and you raise your expectations it is important to provide more powerful reinforcers. Otherwise, regression is more likely to occur.

11. Evaluate The Timing Of Reinforcement

Make sure the awarding of the reinforcer does not break the momentum. Conversely, make sure the reinforcer is not so delayed as to reduce the effectiveness. To avoid this possibility you can use a verbal bridge (e.g., acknowledge the behavior instead of providing reinforcement) as well as nonverbal behavior (e.g., smile, nod, thumbs-up). Work toward eliciting a cluster of responses before giving a tangible reward. Another means of bridging the delay between occurrence of behavior and delivery of the reinforcer is to use a token system or other symbolic representation of the reward the child is earning.

12. In Early Teaching, label The Behavior That Is Being Reinforced

This helps your child to understand the behavior that is being reinforced and that you would like him to repeat. It also strengthens the connection between the reinforcer and the behavior. Labeling the behavior serves as a prompt for yourself as the teacher, keeping you focused on the purpose of trials. Later on it will be less important to specifically label the behavior because your child will be able to understand the contingencies.

13. Over Time, Move To Reinforcement That Is Less Extravagant And More Practical

By using practical and natural reinforcers you enhance generalization. Otherwise, it is likely that when your child participates in more natural settings and reinforcers are not available, his appropriate behaviors will extinguish and disruptive behavior will return.

14. Do Not Use Rewards As Bribery!!!

Do not get you child accustomed to hearing in advance about the reinforcer he will earn. When disruptive behavior occurs, do not remind your child of the reinforcer that he would receive if he stopped or threaten him with its loss. Do not "up the reinforcer ante" following the occurrence of disruptive behavior, i.e., when behavior escalates, do not introduce an additional reinforcer that was not present prior to the escalation.

Bribery is extremely seductive! It looks extremely effective over the short term. Children often immediately stop the disruptive behavior when offered a bribe. This is a short-term strategy that may bring immediate relief but cause lasting problems. You and they can become dependent upon bribery. You will find yourself having to often "remind" them about the reinforcer and what they should be doing to earn it. It also invites negotiation and bargaining, and it could get them into a pattern of first thinking about whether the reinforcer is worth the effort you are asking them to make!

It is preferable to announce the reward **AFTER** the **APPROPRIATE** behavior occurs. Beside countering the disadvantages of bribery, it makes reinforcement less predictable, thereby allowing you to fade reinforcement. Once you begin relying on "If . . . then" bargaining, you admit that the result of this interaction is more important than the process. "If you stop screaming, I will get you a soda." At that point your child will only change his behavior because of what you have offered instead of doing it because he is a child that listens or because it is the right thing to do. This situation focuses upon the external rewards and reduces the chances the child will internalize the desire to make better choices.

15.   Utilize Differential Reinforcement

Perhaps one of the most important methods of teaching skills and modifying disruptive behaviors is differential reinforcement. The concept is simple: provide the strongest reinforcers for the best behaviors or performance. The most desired behaviors get the "to die for" reinforcers while lesser behaviors get a lower quality of reinforcer.

The following chart provides examples of differential reinforcement that may be used in formal therapy:

DIFFERENTIAL AND INFORMATIONAL FEEDBACK

CORRECT & GOOD ATTENDING	CORRECT BUT POOR ATTENDING	INCORRECT BUT GOOD ATTENDING	NO RESPONSE OR INCORRECT WITH POOR ATTENDING
WOW	THAT'S RIGHT	GOOD TRY, BUT...	YOU NEED TO PAY ATTENTION
BEAUTIFUL	CORRECT	ALMOST	YOU NEED TO LISTEN
YOU GOT IT!!!	OK	USE BOTH HANDS	NO
GREAT LISTENING	YEAH	DO IT WHEN I DO IT	WAKE-UP
PERFECT	YOU CAN DO IT BETTER	LET'S TRY IT AGAIN	YOU'RE NOT LISTENING
YOU FIGURED IT OUT	YEP	YOU'RE GETTING CLOSE	YOU'RE NOT PAYING ATTENTION
YOU'RE SO SMART	GOOD	CLOSE, BUT...	YOU NEED TO TRY
TERRIFIC	ALL RIGHT	"THAT'S NOT THE ..."	LISTEN!!!
GOOD GOING	MMM-HUMM	UH-UH	PAY ATTENTION!!!
ALL RIGHT!!!	PRETTY GOOD	NOPE	I'M ASKING YOU A QUESTION
SUPER JOB	GOOD JOB, BUT...	NOT QUITE	YOU NEED TO ANSWER
THAT'S WONDERFUL	THAT'S NICE	SHAKE HEAD NO	HELLO!!!

TONE OF VOICE, FACIAL EXPRESSION AND USE OF TANGIBLE REINFORCERS WILL FURTHER CLARIFY REINFORCER.

Disruptive Behaviors

Disruptive behaviors are perhaps one of the most profound obstacles in treatment. Such behaviors can be extremely difficult to alter, and can create tremendous stress and frustration for everyone. Perhaps the greatest obstacle, however, is everyone's reluctance to address disruptive behaviors. Often they are not even targeted.

There appears to be a number of reasons why programs do not address this critical area. For starters, disruptive behaviors are extremely difficult to change. These behaviors have been extraordinarily effective in your child's learning to adapt and cope with the world. Like any behavior that is adaptive and that has been effective historically, be it one year or ten years, it is extremely difficult to change.

When you attempt to alter disruptive behaviors, you can expect that the intensity and rate of the behavior will increase, sometimes at an alarming rate. Children get upset when we try to take away behaviors that have been very functional for them. Also, they know from past experience that escalating behavior, at least at times, results in people giving in and giving up. Since we do not want to have our children upset and we do not want to bear the brunt of their anger, it is tempting to surrender. This is an all too natural response to such situations. Unfortunately, giving in only serves to reinforce the disruptive behavior, thereby making it far more difficult to change in the future.

Another reason why disruptive behaviors are often overlooked is that people may feel that establishing cognitive skills makes the child seem less disabled. Teaching academic and communication skills is often the area that parents and therapists get most excited about and therefore becomes the focus of intervention. The belief is expressed that without language skills, children's learning opportunities and success in school placement will be greatly reduced.

Ironically, it is the disruptive behavior more than anything else that will actually restrict and even prohibit inclusion. The primary reason for children being removed from such opportunities is the presence of disruptive behaviors, not because of language or social deficits!

Sometimes it is even rationalized that once a child obtains language, his disruptive behaviors will either be eliminated or reduced to manageable levels. Unfortunately, the presence of disruptive behaviors will not only greatly reduce a child's opportunities to learn, but they will greatly slow the pace of learning and negatively affect his or her prognosis. Eventually, it will be necessary to address these behaviors. Unfortunately, with the delay, the behaviors will be even more difficult to address.

Disruptive behaviors are often not even perceived by parents and staff. People can become so accustomed to the behaviors that they are not even aware of behavior being present or not realize how much it is interfering. Often, tremendous accommodations have been made for the child without people being aware of it. Since there is little need for the child to be disruptive, the need to address behavior problems is not apparent. You may only realize that the child is dependent on accommodations you have made when you see his extreme reaction to not being accommodated. Alternatively, adults may have a vague awareness of the possibility of acting out behavior occurring and are motivated by a strong desire to keep peace and therefore subtly adjust their behavior to avoid antagonizing the child.

Behavior problems can also be a lower priority when parents and teachers blindly hope that in time, the behavior will subside on its own. Certainly, the hope is bolstered by the belief that learning new skills such as language, will help in its remission. Unfortunately, this happens all too slowly and resolution of behavior problems is only delayed.

As mentioned earlier, attempting to change disruptive behaviors will often result in your child becoming upset. This is not easy for anyone to experience. Besides not wanting to bear the brunt of his anger, it is extremely distressing to see your child upset. Although the increase in behavior problems is actually a positive sign (i.e., he is aware of the change, he is being interactive, he is demonstrating persistence, etc.) it still does not feel good. You have to remind yourself that the objective is not necessarily to keep children happy in the short run, but to make them happy in the long run. We know how to keep children happy—just let them self-stimulate and give into all their demands. Obviously, this would not be in the child's best interest. As adults, we often need to make decisions that involve curtailing a child's preferences. You have to brush your teeth before you go to bed; you cannot just eat french fries; you cannot throw your toys . . . . Children often would make detrimental choices for themselves and we have a responsibility as adults to ensure that the right decisions are made. This is analogous to getting a shot at the doctor's—it is not pleasant, but it is necessary. We certainly do try to make the experience as positive and pleasant as possible, but recognize that there may be some unavoidable discomfort in the process.

Finally, many people find that dealing with disruptive behaviors takes more patience and skill than teaching something as complex as language. When staff lack these skills, fear and helplessness make it seem easier (in the short run) to simply avoid behavioral issues.

WHEN ARE BEHAVIORS CONSIDERED DETRIMENTAL?

Acting out behaviors such as tantrumming, aggression and noncompliance are easily recognized as disruptive and detrimental. Other behaviors which are passive in nature, such as inattention, not participating, being off-task and isolating may not be disruptive, but nevertheless interfere with development. They are every bit as challenging and essential to address. Although they may not be as obvious, they can be equally, if not more of an obstacle to development. Any behavior that impedes the learning process should be considered as detrimental.

CREATING THE OPTIMAL ENVIRONMENT

Prior to implementing a formal program, it is extremely helpful to create a positive teaching environment. Not only will this greatly enhance the program's effectiveness, but it will make the process more palatable for your child, your family and yourself. This is done by setting up situations where your child is more likely to be calm and cooperative. To start with you should just sit with your child playing with his favorite toy or game while making NO demands. Once he is comfortable with having you there, you can gradually give instructions that are highly likely to be followed. For example, we may say in a very fun but direct tone of voice, "eat the cookie," "watch the video," or "spin the top."

Setting up positive learning situations will not only diminish the disruptive behavior, but will provide the opportunity to reinforce appropriate behavior. Reinforcement, initially, should not only include verbal praise but consist of using tangible rewards such as toys, activities, and food. Verbal praise should include labeling the appropriate behavior. You want to constantly identify the desired behaviors such as "I love how calm you're being," "thanks for listening," "it's great how well you're paying attention." However, you do need to keep the language simple enough for your child to understand.

Besides reducing behavior problems and thereby providing a greater opportunity to reinforce appropriate behaviors there are many other benefits to starting intervention in such a positive manner. First, it allows us to build a positive relationship that is critical for effective therapy. Second, it provides an excellent opportunity to assess strengths and weaknesses. Third, we are able to identify and develop reinforcers. Fourth, it makes the learning situation (i.e., the place, the materials, etc.) something your child will want to come back to. Finally, we can often "sneak" in teaching without eliciting resistive behavior.

ENVIRONMENT AND STRESS

The environment has tremendous effects on behavior. A chaotic setting (i.e., noisy, hot, cluttered, etc.) can lead to behavior outbursts, whereas a more tranquil atmosphere often results in calmer behaviors. This is true for people in general and especially for autistic children. Speaking softly and slowly can often have a tremendously positive impact on disruptive behaviors. The tendency, however, is for people to do just the opposite. They will raise their voice and speak more rapidly. This usually has the effect of not only escalating your child but yourself as well. Also consider how we instinctively react to a child grabbing at materials. Without thinking, we may find ourselves grabbing back to regain control of the materials. However, this type of abrupt physical intervention will have the effect of increasing the chaos and only make the child more frantic in his efforts to control the situation.

It may even be helpful for you to practice stress management techniques yourself, so that you can remain calm in such a situation. By practicing breathing slowly and deeply, reminding yourself to calm down, imagining some pleasant scene or just giving yourself a break, it may help you regain your composure and therefore your child's as well. By remaining calm not only do you reduce the possibility of further agitating the situation but you will most likely increase your objectivity. You will also reduce any negative attention that may reinforce your child's disruptive behaviors.

Reducing potential control battles will also decrease the likelihood of severe disruptive behavior. Giving your child some degree of control by providing choices can be quite effective. Choices such as "would you rather work on the floor or in the chair?", "what would you like to work on?", or "which room would you like to play in?" can often create a calmer situation.

Do not make requests that will lead to battles until you are ready for them (e.g., coming to the chair, eye contact, sitting still, saying hello or goodbye). So you must decide whether it is really important and if you are ready!!! In other words, try to never make requests unless you are prepared to follow through with consequences and perhaps provide physical guidance.

Boredom often contributes to disruptive behaviors. It is necessary to continuously assess how boredom may be contributing to disruptive behaviors. However, we cannot always and do not want to universally eliminate boredom. Children must learn to cope with being bored. But we can certainly attempt not to create needless boredom. The following are some factors you may want to consider in reducing the likelihood of your child being bored or frustrated in therapy:

MAKING THERAPY NATURAL, FUN AND GENERALIZABLE

- Enthusiastic tones
- Varied settings
- Varied instructions (e.g., "What is it?", vs. "What do you see?", vs. "Tell me about this?")
- Interesting, preferred and functional materials
- Do not bore your child by continuing a program that is already mastered
- Do not punish your child for good attending and performance by dragging out tasks when the student is cooperative. Similarly, be careful about shortening programs when fussing occurs
- Maintain a high success rate
- Using your child's preferences (even self-stimulatory objects can be used as reinforcers)
- Intersperse tasks
- Varied and natural reinforcers
- Language should be as natural as possible
- Varied curriculum (e.g., language, play, social, self-help)
- Reduce structure as much as possible (e.g., sometimes work on the floor instead of in the chair)

When disruptive behaviors are exhibited, the least amount of attention necessary should occur. This may mean completely ignoring the behavior. Obviously, if the behavior is danger-ous or extremely disruptive for others (e.g., yelling, swearing, hitting) some attention is unavoid-able as you attempt to stop the behavior (e.g., by removing the child or physically prompting him to put his arms at his side). However, you should do so in a manner that provides as little attention as possible including limiting eye contact and reducing your conversation. Typically, people provide far too much attention. Not only could the attention reinforce the disruptive behavior, but it may also further agitate the child or even serve as an invitation for more disrup-tive behaviors. Even if the procedure would stop the behavior, the child may become highly dependent upon the external control. By providing the least amount of attention, you are avoiding these pitfalls while removing the "payoff" which maintains their disruptive behavior. A full discussion of dealing with disruptive behaviors will follow.

Understanding Disruptive Behaviors

Behavioral programs are based primarily on the assumption that behaviors are learned as a result of their consequences. If a positive consequence follows a behavior, that behavior is more likely to occur in the future. Conversely, a behavior is less likely to occur in the future when a negative consequence follows it. For example, if aggression typically results in an outcome that an individual finds desirable (e.g., attention, avoidance, reduction of frustration, etc.), this person would be more likely to be aggressive in the future. Conversely, if the individual experiences a negative outcome (e.g., having to leave an enjoyable activity), aggression would be less likely to happen next time.

Behavioral interventions which target the decrease of problem behaviors can be divided into two general categories: behavioral enhancement and behavioral reduction strategies. Behavioral reduction programs such as Time-Out, Response Cost, or Extinction are designed to decrease behavior problems by providing a negative environmental consequence contingent on the disruptive behavior. Behavior enhancement procedures like **Differential Reinforcement of Other behavior—DRO, Differential Reinforcement of Incompatible behaviors—DRI,** or **Differential Reinforcement of Lower Rates of behavior—DRL,** are designed to decrease the incidence of disruptive behaviors by reinforcing desirable behaviors and absence of disruptive behavior. Programs often combine behavioral enhancement and reductive procedures. Such programs are designed not only to eliminate disruptive behaviors, but to establish or increase the frequency of appropriate alternative behaviors. This is most effective when the new behaviors being taught evoke naturally reinforcing consequences such as social, play, and communication. Since the child is getting reinforcement through pro-social behavior, he has less inclination to seek the reinforcers he has gotten in the past through disruptive means.

The behavioral approach has been instrumental in the reduction of severely disruptive behaviors such as self-injury, aggression and tantrumming. Moreover, clients who have exhibited deficiencies in communication, play, social, and self-help skills have acquired those critical skills through behavioral interventions.

Although many behavioral interventions have resulted in reductions of disruptive behaviors, the long-term effectiveness of the approach depends on our ability to build in alternative appropriate behavior. Several factors can interfere with the long-term effectiveness of intervention. When programs are designed with a lack of understanding of **WHY** individuals exhibit disruptive behaviors, the underlying factors that maintain disruptive behaviors will not be adequately addressed. Intervention plans all too often assume that all that has to occur is the elimination of a specific maladaptive behavior. Unfortunately, if an individual engages in face slapping because of frustration, for example, stopping the behavior will not be sufficient to eliminate the problem. If the program does not address the client's means of dealing with frustration, it is likely that an alternative behavior, such as head banging, will substitute for the original self-injurious behavior. If a behavior plan is based on a functional analysis of the behavior and therefore addresses the frustration as well as the self-injury, the plan is likely to be far more effective.

The key to effectively changing behaviors over time is to understand the function of the disruptive behavior. One must recognize that disruptive behaviors are not accidental. They serve a purpose. Aggression, for example, may serve the function of reducing stress, avoiding an undesirable task or gaining attention. Disruptive behaviors are adaptive in that they are a way to communicate, impact the environment, and meet one's needs.

Since disruptive behaviors fulfill a need, an effective program must teach your child another behavior that will successfully meet that need. Unless your child is taught an effective alternative behavior to attain his desire, most likely he will develop an equally maladaptive behavior or an old one will eventually return. Your child must be taught, systematically and carefully, a more effective way to get his needs or desires met.

Within the past decade there has been an increased understanding of the nature of disruptive behaviors. However, even with this increased awareness, programs are often inadequately designed and implemented to effectively teach appropriate alternative behaviors. Behavioral programs have shown weaknesses in several areas.

Failure to properly select a replacement behavior is often the first programming difficulty. It may be clear what your child should not do (e.g., not hit others), but it is often more difficult to identify what he *should* do instead. Replacement behavior selection involves not only the analysis of the function of the behavior, but identifying what behavior will effectively serve the same function and what behavior your child is capable of learning. Furthermore, the behavior must be divided into teachable parts (i.e., a task analysis must be conducted). For example, it is not sufficient to merely identify that a stress reduction technique needs to be learned. The specific procedures must be identified (e.g., deep breathing, muscle relaxation, counting, guided imagery, etc.) and a comprehensive and detailed plan must be developed.

Lack of patience is frequently another difficulty in achieving successful programming. It is understandable why everyone would like change to occur rapidly. However, it is not realistic and sometimes not even desirable. Teaching replacement skills is a long process. Disruptive behaviors are generally learned through years of conditioning. Therefore, it is realistic to expect that it may take years for a person to learn new alternative behaviors. Moreover, a systematic and gradual teaching approach is often necessary to fully learn and retain skills. Unfortunately, attempts are often made to teach complex skills all at once. This is not an effective teaching method. One step should be mastered at a time.

The timing of the teaching process is also a common flaw in behavioral interventions. It is important that teaching be conducted under the most optimal conditions possible. That means teaching when your child and the instructor are likely to be most receptive and effective in their actions. This is known as proactive teaching. Typically, the time selected to teach is during or right after the behavior problem occurs. This is absolutely the wrong time for teaching. It is when your child is angry and therefore not receptive to learning and when instructors are frustrated and angry as well and cannot be a positive and patient teachers. It is important to teach at a time when your child is not exhibiting problems and is interested and motivated to learn an alternative behavior.

GUIDELINES FOR DEALING WITH DISRUPTIVE BEHAVIORS

The following are guidelines for you and staff to consider during episodes when disruptive behaviors begin to escalate. Because each situation is different and because everyone has a unique relationship with their child, it would be impossible to specify completely what actions should occur. However, there is a general philosophy that can guide you and certain procedures that should be followed. It is critical, however, to remember that the most effective component of intervention is proactive teaching, which should not occur when your child is agitated.

Acting-out behaviors typically follow a reliable pattern of escalation. That is, disruptive behaviors often progress through stages. The early stage of disruptive behavior is often mild agitation, which may be exhibited through nonverbal behaviors such as pacing, gestures, or irregular breathing, or verbal behaviors such as whining or arguing. If the situation is not resolved or the response is not effective, the behavior will likely proceed to more pronounced acting out, such as property abuse or running away. The final stage may culminate with aggression toward oneself or others.

Each stage typically requires a different response. It is critical to recognize that even the most appropriate response, or one that had been effective in the past may not work consistently. We need to constantly analyze what is currently working and what further teaching is needed.

We must be aware that most children have received many types of intervention. Those strategies may not have been used correctly, consistently or for a long enough duration to be effective. Moreover, commonly used reductive procedures like reprimands, Time-Out, or taking away privileges are generally insufficient by themselves for the long-term reduction of behavior problems. Such strategies are based upon the premise that by providing strong negative conse-

quences, the child will be less likely to act out. Although these procedures may temporarily

interrupt the behavior, they do not address the underlying function of the behavior and may

have the disadvantage of causing undesirable behavioral side effects.

Frequently, people misunderstand behavior reduction procedures. For example, Time-

Out is an intervention which is supposed to entail the child experiencing "Time-Out **FROM**

REINFORCEMENT." In other words, the child should be in a motivating, positive situation

and then when disruptive behaviors occur he would be removed from that setting for a specified

length of time. There are many situations where a child does not find the environment enjoy-

able. So he is quite happy to get out of a situation he does not want to be in. Moreover, when

the child is removed he should not receive any form of reinforcement. However, if you are not

careful when a child is placed in Time-Out (i.e., placed on a chair, in a corner, in the bedroom,

etc.), he may be able to engage in reinforcing behaviors such as self-stimulation. Therefore

Time-Out will actually reinforce or increase the disruptive behavior! As another example,

reprimands can be ineffective because the child may have an emotional reaction or other form

of significant attention in the course of getting a scolding. This attention, although negative,

can still serve to strengthen the disruptive behaviors rather than discourage them.

ESCALATION CYCLE

Children often follow a pattern of escalation. Typically, the disruptive behavior starts

out mild and then builds to a more intense level. The following stages may not be distinct.

Additionally, your child may not follow a reliable escalation pattern. For example, your child

may start out with behaviors that would typically occur in the middle or end phase. It will be

important, therefore, to identify the degree of agitation and the most appropriate response. It is

equally important to use common sense and respond to the uniqueness of the situation.

There are some essential proactive measures that need to be in effect **BEFORE** you get into a crisis situation. One of these is to make certain that you have been giving your child numerous opportunities to make **CHOICES.** By doing this, he will be more accepting of those occasions when choice is not available. Secondly, an ongoing **RICH** schedule of reinforcement is paramount. You will see below that there are occasions when you will need to give out some reinforcement following negative behaviors as the child begins to regain self-control. By arranging it so that **VERY GENEROUS** amounts of reinforcement occur on an ongoing basis when behaviors are normally calm, you can afford to give out a little reinforcement even when his behavior is agitated and still not have to worry about him figuring out that negative behavior is the way to force you to give him some reinforcement. The reason is because the amount of reinforcement he gets for de-escalation is **LESS** than he would have gotten if he had not been disruptive in the first place.

The style you use in these stages is critical. You must remain calm but firm, and emotionally in control. Not only will this help your child remain composed but it will help you retain objectivity and effectiveness. Try to find a way to give choices without having him end up in a situation that is more reinforcing than where you started out. By giving him a modest amount of control, your child may not escalate to extreme disruptiveness.

Having a plan is essential, but that plan must allow for the occurrence of unforeseen behaviors or circumstances. You **MUST** make adjustments **QUICKLY** if your child is having a bad day or if behavior deteriorates.

BEGINNING STAGE

When it seems that your child is beginning to become agitated (as indicated by self-talking, isolating, breathing deeply, etc.) continue with the activity but provide frequent and continuous verbal reinforcement and tangible reinforcement for the appropriate responses. For example, tell your child how well he is doing and time access to stronger reinforcers to coincide with lessening of agitation. This is the basic *de-escalation strategy*. Remember that there must be an ongoing schedule that ensures that the most preferred reinforcers are provided when there is no sign of disruptive behaviors. However, for those situations where his behavior has escalated, you need to have a means of encouraging him to regain self-control. If you withheld all reinforcement, he would have no incentive to turn his behavior around. Fortunately, agitated behavior does not always remain at a constant state. There are natural variations in the intensity of the behavior and occasional pauses. This allows you an opportunity to provide reinforcement during the moments of pause. As longer stretches of calm behavior occur, you should increase the strength of the reinforcement. Make certain, though, that the reinforcement for de-escalation is less than would have occurred if the agitation had not started in the first place.

If there is a surge in the agitation, then you should once again ignore the behavior. **BUT DO NOT IGNORE THE CHILD!** The rationale for remaining with the child at the activity is to make it clear to him that disruptive behaviors will not enable him to get out of tasks. Moreover, if you remove yourself from the situation, you will miss the opportunity to reinforce at the appropriate moments of de-escalation. If you completely ignored the child, his behavior would likely intensify and lead to greater turmoil.

SECOND STAGE

Keep in mind that we often arrive at this more intense level of escalation as a result of ineffective intervention in the first stage or because we misread the behavior. However, there will be times that this happens (we are only human after all!) and there will be times when even the best intervention is not effective in the first stage. If your child does become moderately disruptive (e.g., says "no" loudly, paces, talks loudly to himself, cries, etc.) it may be necessary to employ stimulus change procedures. It is likely that there is something present in the situation that is causing the intensified distress. If you can identify it, then you may be able to change the situation by altering the activity or setting. There are two different kinds of situation that can lead to this more intense level of acting out. One is that the child is simply being manipulative and hoping that this higher level of disruptiveness will convince you that you need to give in. In this case it is very important that whatever the de-escalation procedure, we do not end up with his hope being confirmed. Here you need to be firm and unsympathetic.

A different situation results from our realization that in fact the situation is too demanding for the child and therefore we need to make adjustments. Examples of this might be when we realize we have let the task go on too long, we have not prompted adequately, the task is too difficult, or we have not been giving sufficient reinforcement. In other words, he has good reason to be upset and we need to be sympathetic to that, although he still is not justified in carrying on in an inappropriate manner. The graceful way to resolve such situations is through redirection. The antecedents that are triggering the behavior may be eliminated and thereby reduce acting-out. If at all possible, this should be done in a subtle way, so that your child is less likely to learn that by being disruptive he is able to avoid non-preferred activities. The kind of response that you should be redirecting him to is one that he knows well how to do, and that can be readily prompted if he refuses to attempt them. We often use receptive instructions, nonverbal imitation, or simple motor tasks to reestablish compliant behavior.

As always, provide verbal and tangible reinforcement when your child is calm and appropriate and provide minimal attention when disruptive. You can capitalize on the fact that certain kinds of reinforcer not only have a motivating effect, but they also are soothing and comforting. Examples would be physical comfort, soft voice, hugs, pats and singing. You must be very careful in the timing of the delivery of these reinforcers. If it is only a short time since the disruptive behavior was occurring (about 30 seconds or less) you cannot afford to give very much of this type of reinforcer, because you will also be partially reinforcing the very recent inappropriate behavior. As more time goes by since the child was being disruptive (at least a few minutes), you can give large amounts of soothing reinforcers and you will be mostly reinforcing self-control. You will also get the added effect that the soothing properties of the reinforcers also mean that agitation is being wiped away and therefore the likelihood of re-escalation is drastically reduced.

If the original task is indeed a reasonable one to expect the child to perform, you should attempt to get back to the task and get whatever you think is possible under the circumstances before ending the teaching session. Remember that this is a long term shaping process and you do not have to accomplish everything in this one session. However, you do want to end up at a point which moves you at least somewhat closer to that long-term goal.

THIRD STAGE

When your child is becoming extremely agitated (e.g., flailing and combative, screaming, throwing objects, hitting others, self-injury, etc.) it is usually necessary to become quite firm and structured. If you have previously worked on establishing instructional control (e.g., hands down) this can be an effective means of counteracting the disruptive behavior. Try to give instructions that are as specific as possible, stating clearly and in a firm tone of voice what it **IS** that needs to be done rather than what **NOT** to do, for example, "you need to sit in the chair").

However, you may not always be able to think of just the right thing to say and often providing instructions to "stop it" may help regain control. Be sure to make such statements only once or twice or they will lose their effectiveness, you lose credibility, and the situation becomes more chaotic. Provide verbal and tangible reinforcement for any signs of de-escalation and provide as little attention as possible for the disruptive behaviors.

Threats are something that staff are often tempted to resort to. One reason why they do this is that they may indeed result in a fairly immediate cessation of behavior. The problem is that using such heavy-handed means of controlling behavior usually leads to worsening of behavior at other times. Reliance on threats to control behavior results in a pattern of behavior where children learn to respond only to directives that are accompanied by strongly worded consequences and ignore directives that are given in an ordinary, straightforward manner. The long-term goal should be for the child to learn that consequences, both positive and negative are certain to occur, regardless of whether they are being verbalized. Also, you are at a disadvantage when you have committed yourself to a specific consequence in advance. It is better to let the child worry about what the consequence might be. That way, you give yourself more time to make the appropriate decision about any consequence that may be necessary.

Whatever the consequence, it should be implemented by the person who was working with the child at the time the behavior happened. Turning control of the child over to a "higher authority" only undermines the role of the person who is deferring. In effect, you are saying to the child, "I can't control your behavior, so I need to turn to this other person." Finally, **YOU SHOULD NEVER THREATEN SOMETHING THAT YOU WOULD NOT ACTUALLY BE PREPARED TO CARRY OUT OR THAT WOULD BE INAPPROPRIATE (e.g., "I'm going to lock you in your room and never let you out!").**

As the child is showing better ability to control himself, you can remind him that he will be earning a reinforcer (specified or unspecified) now that he is calm and doing good work. Just be careful that this does not turn into bribery, and that it should be used only as a last resort in order to avoid having to use hands-on procedures.

FINAL STAGE

If you feel your child poses a danger to himself or others, then it is necessary to utilize Management of Assaultive Behavior (MAB) or other hands-on procedures including escorts or containment. For example, MAB procedures would be used if severe self-injury is occurring. Naturally, there should be as little attention as possible, and you should monitor closely for the moment when your child's behavior starts to de-escalate so that you can immediately reinforce both verbally, and with tangibles.

**HANDS-ON PROCEDURES SHOULD ONLY BE USED WHEN YOU HAVE
EXHAUSTED OTHER MEANS AND THE SITUATION HAS
THE POTENTIAL OF BECOMING DANGEROUS.**

ALL STAGES

Be sensitive to how your child responds to praise or reinforcement when provided during the cycle. Frequently, children either reject such interventions or escalate in response to them. Your child will let you know through his behavior if your reinforcement is effective. If calm, relaxed or less agitated behavior is observed, your reinforcers are effective.

If agitation increases or the child throws or rejects the tangible reinforcer you provided, it is time to reconsider your choice of reward. Frequently, children whose behavior escalates when reinforcement or feedback is provided have a high need for control or power in the environment. Some strategies to try, include not commenting directly on the behavior. For example, instead of saying "I like how calm you are", try something like "You are nice to be with" or comment to the child regarding something he is doing (e.g., "Do you want to look at this book with me?")

This may provide attention without directly focusing on the disruptive behavior. If you wish to use a tangible reward and it is rejected, try to simply place it near your child and end the need for him to accept it from your hands. This rewards him for calm behavior and allows him to retain some control in the situation. It would appear that for some children taking a reward from a person directly places them in a one-down position and further frustrates them.

Once the agitation has subsided, record the event. Not only does this provide an account of the event, but will help to analyze the pattern of escalation and the effectiveness of the intervention and therefore help to identify what modifications are required. The data you keep on the frequency and intensity of the behavior will provide a reliable means of determining whether the intervention is working.

SPECIFIC BEHAVIOR MANAGEMENT TECHNIQUES

Even the most effective behavior management program will not guarantee complete elimination of disruptive behaviors. The addition of teaching appropriate alternative behaviors, effective reinforcement procedures, and creating the optimal environment will, however, bring you much closer to that goal. The following are specific guidelines to maximize effectiveness of behavioral interventions:

1.   As discussed previously, you want to provide the least amount of attention necessary whenever disruptive behaviors are exhibited. Attention and other forms of reinforcement should occur in the absence of the disruptive behavior. You must be extremely careful that the occurrence of disruptive behaviors does not become a cue for you to increase reinforcement. Otherwise, your child will engage in disruptive behaviors so that when he stops, he will receive reinforcement. The best way to guard against this is to maintain a rich schedule of reinforcement prior to the onset of disruptive behaviors.

Also, make sure that the amount of reinforcement given for de-escalation is less than he would otherwise have gotten.

2.   Reinforcing de-escalation is extremely important. All too often, people wait until the child is completely calm before providing reinforcement. This may take too long and only serves to further escalate the behavior. Do not wait until disruptive behaviors have been eliminated. Reinforce slight reductions in disruptive behavior. Avoid the control battle and give the child a way to save face and rejoin the environment calmly. Be sure to praise him and label the de-escalation (e.g., "You're showing really good control; I love how you are calming down").

3.   You may need to use **SUBTLE** redirection procedures. The subtler the redirection, the less likely he will sense that he has gotten out of something. It is important to try and return to the original task and bring it to a successful conclusion. Try to be as least intrusive as possible, so that he does not become dependent on the staff to maintain control **FOR** him. Intrusive prompting and instructions are very difficult to fade. Less directive procedures will promote internalization of self-control steps.

4.   Response prevention is a procedure that is often used with behaviors such as self-stimulation and low-level aggression or self-abuse. If this is the approach to be used, then you must stop the behavior as quickly as possible, using the least amount of attention. Normally, we give a neutral physical prompt and do not comment about it. This is done without interrupting the task or activity which the child receives reinforcement for continuing to perform.

5.   Creating "Behavioral Momentum" is a powerful strategy for counteracting disruptive behavior or inattention. When your child is listening and behaving well, the probability of disruptive behaviors occurring is greatly diminished. By creating a pattern of success,

you are building momentum. For example, if you start therapy with play activities or highly preferred tasks, your child is more likely to behave. Once you are into tasks, if behavior deteriorates, accelerated prompting followed by moderate reinforcers will help to restore momentum. As discussed previously, a calm and positive environment is important as well.

6.   Implementing Stress Management and Errorless Compliance training programs are essential in reducing disruptive behaviors as well as creating an optimal environment. These programs will be discussed later.

7.   Remember that the most important thing is what you do **BEFORE** the disruptive behavior occurs to keep it from happening. Two of the most useful guidelines on the preventive use of positive reinforcement:

> *"Catch your child being good."*

> *"Praise the best; ignore the rest."*

Behavior Programs

DISRUPTIVE BEHAVIORS

Your child's disruptive behaviors, such as crying, tantrumming, and aggression, most likely serve multiple functions. Reduction of frustration and stress is often a primary function of disruptive behaviors. Behaviors may also be avoidance-related. That is, children are often able to avoid non-preferred situations through engaging in disruptive behaviors. Another purpose of acting-out may be the attention received following such behavior.

Since frustration is a likely factor in triggering disruptive behaviors, a program designed to increase your child's tolerance to non-preferred situations needs to be implemented. Your child will need to learn to cope with unpleasant situations. Through gradual exposure to non-preferred situations, frustration tolerance will be gradually increased. Moreover, your child will learn that disruptive behavior will not result in avoidance. It will be important that your child receives minimal attention for disruptive behaviors so as not to provide an incentive for acting out.

The program will first involve identifying events that are frustrating for your child. Parent and teacher observations will be critical in identifying such stressors. Additionally, a review of data and reports may also reveal situations that trigger acting-out. Denial of desires, non-preferred situations, changes in routines or not receiving reinforcers are likely stressors.

Frustrating situations then should be categorized into at least three distinct levels. Level 1's will be those that are only mildly agitating, whereas level 3's will be reserved for events that provoke tremendous agitation. Level 2 will be for events in between. Naturally, you can create more than three levels. Obviously, stressors can change. That is, what was mildly annoying yesterday may create tremendous anger today!

The next step involves creating a relaxation response for your child. Typically, we will have a child sit in a very comfortable chair. The lights will be dimmed and relaxing music is played. In an extremely relaxing voice (i.e., slow and soft) we will instruct the child to calm. We closely observe the child and label and praise him for becoming relaxed. These sessions will continue for as long as it is necessary for him to learn to become relaxed.

Once he has learned to relax, it is time to start exposing him to the stressors. We start with one stressor from the mild category. We attempt to select the one that is the mildest. Once the child is extremely relaxed, he is exposed for a short amount of time to the situation. Extensive reinforcement is provided for remaining calm. Then the stressor is reintroduced. Once again, reinforcement is provided for calmness. Sessions are repeated until your child is able to remain calm to the first stressor for approximately five teaching sessions.

Once your child has successfully mastered the first stressor, exposure to the second stressor will occur. The program will continue until he has been exposed to all the steps in the hierarchy. Additionally, your child will be gradually and systematically exposed to situations in the natural environment.

Since it will not be possible to neutralize all upsetting events, eventually your child should be trained in relaxation procedures as a management response to mildly stressful occurrences. Several procedures should be tested in order to identify the most effective procedure. Stress management procedures such as tensing and then releasing, listening to music, deep breathing, guided imagery should be attempted. Once identified, the selected techniques are taught and then utilization is prompted and reinforced as an alternative management response to stress. As your child's language develops, simple verbal expression of emotions, in response to stress may eventually be added to his coping repertoire.

FRUSTRATION TOLERANCE PROGRAM

Phase 1

1. Identify situations that are stressful to the child (by asking parents and teachers, observing the child, noting the pattern of disruptive behavior).

2. Arrange situations in a hierarchy from least to most stressful.

Phase 2

1. While the child is as relaxed as possible (i.e., sitting in comfortable chair, dimmed lights, soft music) expose him to the least stressful situation contained in the hierarchy.

2. Provide praise and intermittent reinforcement contingent upon calm behavior. It may be necessary to gradually shape more appropriate responding.

3. Gradually move the teaching to more natural environments and situations.

4. When he exhibits calm behaviors to the least stressful situation for five consecutive teaching sessions, move to the next level of stress.

5. Proceed through the hierarchy.

Phase 3

1. Teach the child relaxation procedures.

2. Once he has learned relaxation techniques, prompt him to use the procedures when minimally stressed.

3. Fade prompt as rapidly as possible.

STRESS HIERARCHY

Mildly Annoying	Moderately Annoying	Extremely Annoying
_____	_____	_____
_____	_____	_____
_____	_____	_____
_____	_____	_____
_____	_____	_____
_____	_____	_____
_____	_____	_____
_____	_____	_____
_____	_____	_____
_____	_____	_____
_____	_____	_____
_____	_____	_____
_____	_____	_____
_____	_____	_____
_____	_____	_____
_____	_____	_____
_____	_____	_____
_____	_____	_____
_____	_____	_____

NONCOMPLIANCE

The compliance program is based upon facilitating your child's successful following of instructions by gradually increasing demands. Initially your child will only be asked to complete tasks that he finds highly preferable. For example, your child may be asked to eat a snack, play with a favorite toy, or even self-stimulate. Issuing such instructions will most likely result in compliance, thereby providing an opportunity to praise and reward following instructions. Gradually, the instructions will be a little less desirable while maintaining extensive reinforcement for compliance.

POINTERS TO FACILITATE COMPLIANCE

1.   Only issue instructions with which you are willing to follow through. Following through requires either motoring your child through task or providing a meaningful consequence for compliance. As your child ages, motoring through should be kept to a minimum.

2.   Do not issue multiple instructions in a short time span (e.g., three instructions in 10 seconds). Otherwise, you will promote noncompliance as well as create an agitating situation.

3.   Provide your child positive choices (e.g., "Do you want to go outside and play or would you like to watch a video?).

4.   Also provide your child forced choices (e.g., "Do you want to take a bath or do you want to go to bed?").

5.   When your child does not follow instructions, you should be as neutral as possible.

6.   Attempt to facilitate your child's compliance by "sandwiching" non-preferred tasks between easier tasks. Making tasks fun sets up the environment to facilitate compliance.

7.   Catch your child listening. For example, when your child is about to close the door, say "Please close the door" and then reinforce him for cooperating.

8.   Issue instructions calmly with the expectation that your child will listen.

9.   Provide your child with areas of control.

10.   **GIVE YOUR CHILD MEANINGFUL REINFORCERS WHEN LISTENING OCCURS.**

COMPLIANCE PROGRAM

Phase 1

1.   Identify instructions that are typically issued at home.

2.   Determine the rate of compliance to the various instructions.

3.   Construct a hierarchy of instructions, ranging from those with the highest probability of compliance (e.g., "Eat the cookie.") to those with lower probability of compliance (e.g., "Give your brother his toy back.").

Phase 2

1.   The teacher will issue the requests with the highest probability of compliance.

2.   Reinforcement will be provided upon compliance with these requests.

3.   When your child exhibits compliance for three consecutive sessions, move to the next phase.

Phase 3

1.   The teacher will issue requests with a high probability of compliance and a few requests with a lower probability of compliance.

2.   Reinforcement will be provided upon compliance with the requests.

3.   When your child exhibits compliance for three consecutive sessions, move to the next phase.

Remaining Phases

1.   Increasingly, requests to complete non-preferred tasks will be gradually introduced while requests to complete preferred tasks will be reduced.

COMPLIANCE HIERARCHY

SORT INSTRUCTIONS TYPICALLY PROVIDED THROUGHOUT THE DAY INTO THE FOLLOWING CATEGORIES:

	ALWAYS (e.g. 100%)	OFTEN (e.g., 75%)	SOMETIMES (e.g., 50%)	RARELY (e.g., 25%)	NEVER (e.g., 0%)
1.	_____	_____	_____	_____	_____
2.	_____	_____	_____	_____	_____
3.	_____	_____	_____	_____	_____
4.	_____	_____	_____	_____	_____
5.	_____	_____	_____	_____	_____
6.	_____	_____	_____	_____	_____
7.	_____	_____	_____	_____	_____
8.	_____	_____	_____	_____	_____
9.	_____	_____	_____	_____	_____
10.	_____	_____	_____	_____	_____
11.	_____	_____	_____	_____	_____
12.	_____	_____	_____	_____	_____
13.	_____	_____	_____	_____	_____
14.	_____	_____	_____	_____	_____
15.	_____	_____	_____	_____	_____
16.	_____	_____	_____	_____	_____
17.	_____	_____	_____	_____	_____
18.	_____	_____	_____	_____	_____
19.	_____	_____	_____	_____	_____
20.	_____	_____	_____	_____	_____

REACTIVE PROGRAM - POSITIVE

Phase 1
1. Your child will be provided with verbal praise every five minutes for the absence of maladaptive behaviors

2. After three consecutive periods of the absence of maladaptive behaviors, your child will be provided a reinforcer and verbal praise

Phase 2
1. Your child will be provided verbal praise every fifteen minutes for the absence of maladaptive behaviors

2. After three consecutive periods of the absence of maladaptive behaviors, your child will be provided a reinforcer and verbal praise

Phase 3
1. Your child will be provided verbal praise every 30 minutes for the absence of maladaptive behaviors

2. After two consecutive periods of the absence of maladaptive behaviors, your child will be provided a reinforcer and verbal praise

Remaining Phases
Gradually increase the duration of time required to receive reinforcement. Once your child has reached this phase, your child may be allowed certain reinforcers as often as desired (within reason), as long as no maladaptive behaviors have occurred for the preceding two hours.

REACTIVE PROGRAM - REDUCTIVE

1. Your child will lose the opportunity to receive scheduled verbal reinforcement and the tangible reinforcer when specified undesired behaviors occur

2. Attention will be kept to a minimum upon the occurrence of specified undesired behaviors

Self-Stimulatory Behaviors

Self-stimulatory behavior is one of the major diagnostic features of autism. Self-stimulation is repetitive, stereotyped behavior that does not appear to serve any other function beyond sensory gratification. There are three reasons why we would target self-stimulation for reduction: 1) it greatly interferes with attention; 2) it is highly reinforcing to the child and makes other, more adaptive reinforcers less appealing; 3) it is stigmatizing. When an individual engages in self-stimulation, his attention is usually fully engaged in the behavior and the person does not process important information. This greatly interferes with learning. Because self-stimulation is so reinforcing to the individual, it is often difficult to motivate him to decrease the behavior.

Self-stimulation can involve any of the five senses as well as proprioception and takes many forms. Body movement is one of the major categories. This includes rocking, hand flapping, twirling oneself. Hand regarding also involves body movement but has an additional component that is visual. Gazing is more of a pure form of visual self-stimulation, as is watching things move across visual lines, such as looking through the slats of a fence.

A second category of self-stimulation is using objects for the primary purpose of providing sensory input. Examples commonly observed include flapping objects such as paper and leaves, twirling string between the fingertips, spinning objects, turning wheels of a car, sifting sand, splashing water and picking lint. When an autistic child is interacting with a toy it may appear as though he is actually playing. However, you will often see that the toy is not being used in its intended fashion, such as spinning the wheels of the car instead of "driving" the car. Repetitive use of objects such as tapping would also fit in this category.

A third type of self-stimulation is rituals and obsessions. These can be quite varied. Lining up objects, holding items, wearing the same clothes, insisting that things not be moved (e.g., furniture), talking over and over about certain topics (verbal perseveration), closing doors, and problems with transitions are common examples. These often involve rules that the child has developed and insists on following as well as trying to get other people to follow the rules. As with obsessional behavior, these rules greatly interfere with activities of daily life. Also like obsessions, they often get stronger and more ingrained with time, and the child becomes more resistant to altering the obsession.

When bored, most people will engage in various forms of self-stimulation, be it day-dreaming or tapping their foot, twirling their hair or playing with a pencil. The difference, however, is that the typical person is able to continue attending and the self-stimulatory behavior is usually more subtle (i.e., less repetitious and not as inappropriate looking). Most important this is not the only, or the most desired means of receiving gratification. Most people receive greater satisfaction through recreation, hobbies and their connection with others. Also, most people can refrain from self-stimulation in order to avoid negative social reactions. For example, we do not pick our teeth when people are watching.

Self-stimulatory behaviors in autistic children may occur continuously or in situations that are boring or stressful. Besides looking inappropriate, the child's ability to attend while engaged is self-stimulation is drastically reduced. Often children are suspected of being visually and hearing impaired because of this total lack of responding. There may even be a raised threshold for experiencing pain because self-stimulation is blocking out the intensity of the sensation.

Self-stimulation is similar to addictive behaviors. The drive to engage in self-stimulatory activity can result in behaviors that resemble a drug induced state. As long as the individual is "high" or preoccupied with getting the "high," he will not learn. Similarly, the addiction gets worse and feeds on itself! Valuable learning opportunities are lost and, like other addicts, the child experiences further arrested development as withdrawal into oneself becomes more pronounced. It is critical to seize control over this behavior. There are several strategies that can be used to reduce and hopefully eliminate its interfering qualities.

FUNCTIONS OF SELF-STIMULATION

As discussed in the section on "Disruptive Behaviors," self-stimulation, like all disruptive behavior, potentially serves multiple purposes. As the name implies, the primary function these behaviors generally serve is to provide self-stimulation. People with autism often do not find people or the environment interesting. Engaging in these behaviors is an extremely adaptive means of receiving gratification. Consequently, when bored or simply unoccupied, they will exhibit self-stimulation. Whereas most children will often play with toys or seek out others (e.g., parents, sibling, peers, etc.), individuals with autism often prefer to engage in self-stimulation.

A second possible function of self-stimulation is to reduce frustration and stress. For example, during transitions, in chaotic situations, or during incorrect responding, self-stimulation will often be observed. The behavior appears to serve the purpose of soothing oneself as well as blocking out the source of frustration. It also may serve as a signal for others to reduce demands or provide assistance by removing the source of frustration. Thus, self-stimulation should be viewed as adaptive from the child's perspective and extremely rewarding.

Over time, self-stimulation becomes more and more powerful. Therefore, it becomes extremely difficult to contain and suppress. In younger children, elimination of the behavior may be a realistic goal, but with older children, reduction may have to be the objective. Both age groups can benefit from shaping self-stimulation into more age-typical behaviors. Naturally, the earlier intervention can occur, the more successful the outcome.

As with any behavior problem, there are several strategies that can be employed. As discussed previously, behavior management procedures can be separated into "**Proactive**" and "**Reactive**" strategies. The most effective approach is a combination of both. The proactive strategies will teach alternative replacement behaviors that are designed to provide the individual satisfaction similar to the self-stimulation. Reactive methods will be designed to reduce the self-stimulation by reducing or even eliminating the reinforcement, building in response cost, and providing reinforcement for alternative behaviors.

REACTIVE PROCEDURES

SYSTEMATIC IGNORING

Usually, self-stimulation provides its own source of reinforcement. Your child would most likely be quite happy to have you ignore him, so he can engage in self-stimulation without any distractions. Any interference in the behavior would be most unappreciated because you would be depriving him of the stimulation he enjoys. People sometimes equate ignoring with extinction. However, since the reinforcer in this case has little to do with attention, systematic ignoring rarely is effective in reducing or eliminating the behavior. Similarly, Time-Out is also generally very ineffective. Time-Out's effectiveness is dependent upon the child being removed from a rewarding activity or environment. However, since Time-Out actually provides the ideal opportunity to self-stimulate, the procedure may actually lead to an increase in self-stimulation.

REINFORCEMENT

As with all behavior problems, the use of reinforcement procedures to reduce self-stimulation is vital. There are several reinforcement procedures that may be appropriate. Differential Reinforcement of Incompatible/Alternative Behaviors (DRI/DRA), Differential Reinforcement of Other Behaviors (DRO) and Differential Reinforcement of Lower Rates of Behaviors (DRL) are examples of reinforcement procedures that will provide reinforcement and motivate the child to engage in behaviors other than self-stimulation. Any reductive program **MUST BE** used in conjunction with some type of a differential reinforcement program.

RESPONSE PREVENTION

Stopping the behavior immediately, whenever it occurs, will reduce or even eliminate the reinforcement. Since the behavior itself provides its own reinforcement, every second one is engaged in self-stimulation, one is receiving reinforcement. It is similar to feeding oneself candy! The faster the behavior is blocked, the less time the child spends self-delivering reinforcement.

The way you stop the behavior is extremely important. As with most behaviors, you should use the least directive method that will stop the behavior. The following is a hierarchy of methods ranging from least to most directive:

LESS DIRECTIVE						**MORE DIRECTIVE**
PAUSE	GLANCE	FACIAL EXPRESSION	GESTURE	PARTIAL PHYSICAL	FULL PHYSICAL	VERBAL

The rationale for using the least directive method is similar to the reason why you use the least directive prompts, namely, that it is easier to fade the intervention. Using verbal reminders or reprimands is generally more difficult to fade than using gestures. The more indirect the procedure, the more likely the child will internalize, and the less likely it will be necessary to use external control procedures. The less perceptible the intervention, the less the child's response is externalized. For example, a subtle touch may stop the behavior without him even being aware of your touch. Although self-stimulation is not attention motivated, it is important that it does not become partially or secondarily motivated by attention. Therefore, using the least directive method will reduce the possibility of attention reinforcing this behavior.

Please note that directiveness does not necessarily equate to intrusiveness. Intrusiveness entails an impingement upon the child's freedom. For example, verbal redirection does not involve any physical force and therefore might be thought of as less intrusive. However, verbal prompts are often more difficult to fade and therefore do not lead as readily to independence. Verbal prompts should only be used when the child is confused or needs information about what behavior is expected. Once he understands the concept or expected behavior, nonspecific prompts should be used. A nonspecific prompt is a "get going" cue that does not tell the child what specifically to do.

There are important reasons for using the least intrusive method as well as the least directive. First, it reduces the likelihood of a power struggle. Often when intrusive methods are used, it incites resistance and a child may be provoked to extreme measures to win the battle. Secondly, using nonintrusive procedures is also extremely important in not calling others' attention to what is occurring. When working in an inclusive situation such as in a classroom, at the park or in the community, one would always prefer to call the least amount of attention to the child so as not to identify or stigmatize the child.

Remember that it is critical to stop the behavior as soon as it is observed. It is best if you can stop it before it even occurs, breaking the cycle at its onset. Initially, therefore, you may need to use a more intrusive procedure, such as a physical prompt because a subtler procedure will not stop the behavior. Naturally, however, the goal is to quickly fade to a less directive procedure. Once you stop the behavior, direct your child to a more appropriate activity. As he begins exhibiting appropriate behavior, provide appropriate reinforcement. As more time goes by with the exhibition of appropriate behavior, the reinforcement should be increased.

REDUCING THE REINFORCING VALUE OF SELF-STIMULATION

There are several strategies that can be used to alter the satisfaction your child may receive through self-stimulation. One procedure shown to be effective in reducing self-stimulation is actually using self-stimulation as a reinforcer. Although this may not seem sensible, it can actually serve two purposes. Not only will it serve as a powerful reinforcer, but it will gradually reduce the gratification your child receives from the behavior.

First, you can provide a limited opportunity to self-stimulate as a reward for the occurrence of certain desired behaviors or even the absence of self-stimulation. Therefore, you are actually using the self-stimulation to develop appropriate alternative behaviors to take its place. Besides the advantage of developing a replacement behavior, there is a more important effect of using this procedure. You are actually changing the nature of the behavior. Self-stimulation by its very character is internally controlled by the child. When you establish a contingency, you are taking control of the behavior, subtly altering it, placing limits and conditions on it. By moving the behavior from internal to external control, you have created the effect of reducing its reinforcing value. Gradually, you can contain the behavior and slowly reduce it by requiring longer periods of not self-stimulating in order to receive reinforcement.

Another way to reduce the reinforcement value of self-stimulation is to orchestrate situations so your child chooses not to self-stimulate. For example, give him the choice between eating his very favorite food or watching his favorite cartoon or self-stimulating. Naturally, you cannot use this approach effectively unless you have established alternatives that he will find more desirable. By choosing not to engage in self-stimulation, he is himself reducing the positive value of his own self-stimulation.

STIMULUS CONTROL

Stimulus control procedures are designed with the intent of creating environments and/ or situations that do not elicit the self-stimulatory behaviors. This may be accomplished by establishing rooms in your house or times of the day when this behavior is not allowed to occur. By permitting it to occur only under limited conditions, you will be limiting it to more acceptable circumstances as well as reducing its rate. Your goal may be to continue reducing it until it is eliminated. For example, you may initially establish the rule that it can only occur in the bedroom and family room and then subsequently limit it to only the bedroom. Similarly, you may limit its occurrence to only certain times during the day and gradually reduce the time periods when it is permitted.

PROACTIVE PROCEDURES

The most important part of an effective plan for any behavior is teaching appropriate alternatives. This is usually a long and tedious process filled with frustrations. However, without your child learning appropriate alternative behaviors, it is unlikely that you will achieve long-term success. Even the strongest reactive program by itself is unlikely to reduce behavior problems. Simply eliminating the behavior does not provide an alternative means for your child to fulfill the function that the disruptive behavior has filled. You must teach appropriate alternative behaviors. Otherwise self-stimulation will return or another inappropriate behavior will most likely develop.

Identifying the replacement behavior is based upon identifying the function of the self-stimulatory behavior. Because self-stimulation is typically a means to receive certain types of sensory input, teaching play, recreation and interactional skills that have strong sensory components will be the most effective way to establish replacement behaviors. Your child must learn skills that will lead to gratification so he will not need to engage in self-stimulation in order to be entertained.

Self-stimulation most likely serves other functions as well, thereby necessitating the teaching of additional skills. Teaching your child appropriate ways to cope with frustration may also be necessary in order to reduce self-stimulation. By reducing frustration, you may reduce situations where self-stimulation occurs. Communication skills may also be an effective deterrent to self-stimulation. For example, some children self-stimulate when they do not know how to respond. By teaching them to indicate they do not know an answer or are confused, through verbal on nonverbal communication means, there may be less need to engage in self-stimulation.

PROGRAMS DESIGNED SPECIFICALLY TO TEACH PLAY, SOCIAL AND COMMUNICATION SKILLS ARE DESCRIBED EXTENSIVELY IN OTHER SECTIONS

PRACTICALITY

Reducing self-stimulation will be one of your greatest challenges. It is extremely powerful, interfering behavior that your child most likely finds more reinforcing than any other activity. Attempting to eliminate it throughout the day will most likely be an impossible task. Although reducing self-stimulation is important, setting yourself up to do something so difficult will most likely create tremendous stress in you and your family. Therefore, your ability to implement any behavior program effectively will be greatly diminished.

It is always preferable to run a program with precision for a shorter length of time rather than inconsistently for a greater length of time. Therefore, it is highly recommended that you identify how long and under what conditions you can follow the program. Your child will eventually learn the situations when the behavior is not accepted. Naturally, he will also learn that at other times he can engage in self-stimulation. As you effectively gain control over self-stimulation you need to increase the time and circumstances during which you intervene. You might wish to be able to completely eliminate self-stimulation from the outset but the best approach to take is one that will be successful for both you and your child. **MORE IS NOT NECESSARILY BETTER!!!**

Sleep Problems

A child who has difficulties going to bed, falling asleep, staying asleep, and returning to sleep, can make nighttime a horrible ordeal. Parents' patience can often be tested through long hours of frustration before their child goes to sleep. In the end, parents often find themselves in the predicament of either sleeping in their child's bed or having the child sleep in their bed if anyone is to get some sleep.

Sleep disturbances place a tremendous strain on the entire family. Brother's and Sister's sleep is often disturbed as a result of the battle over bedtime. Parents rarely get a good night's sleep, which saps their much-needed energy for the next day. Without restful sleep, your child's ability to learn new and critical skills is greatly decreased. Obviously, with a tired child, therapy will be greatly affected.

As we all know, sleep habits are extremely difficult to change. Even for adults, sleeping on a different side of the bed, sleeping with a different pillow, or sleeping in a different bed can disturb sleep. Naturally, once a child is used to going to bed late at night or sleeping with his parents, any change in the routine will be met with resistance. However, the longer you wait, the more ingrained the pattern becomes. We suggest that you address the problem sooner rather than later. Taking the easier solution today will only make the problem harder to solve tomorrow. The only time to consider a delay is when sleeping problems might be more successfully tackled once compliance gains have been achieved in other areas.

Typically, with one week of hard work, everyone will be enjoying a good night's sleep. A warning, however: it will not be an easy week! The program may result in your not sleeping at all during the night for the first several days. We suggest that you prepare yourself by getting as much sleep as you can before you begin the program and once it is underway you should plan to catch up on your sleep during the day. Parents often arrange to have a four-day weekend to begin the program or even wait until their vacation. Parents have also requested assistance from relatives to share the sleepless nights that may be required. Thoroughness in following the program will be essential. Choose a period that you will best be able to provide consistent intervention.

There is a final caveat. If you have been making partial attempts to change nighttime behavior, but have given in after crying or other resistive behavior, your child has been on an intermittent reinforcement schedule: sometimes he gets what he wants, sometimes he does not. He has seen you attempt to be firm but has learned that by escalating his behavior, he can over-come your resolve. This will make it harder for you to achieve your goal the next time you attempt to improve the nighttime routine. As strange as it may sound, you would be better off giving in right away for a week or two before attempting another intervention. That way, when you do start the program, the change from status quo will be more evident to the child and extinction of his disruptive behaviors will not take as long.

ESTABLISHING A NIGHTTIME ROUTINE

The basic premise of the program is to give your child the tools to fall asleep independently, both at the beginning of the night and during the middle of the night. Remember that it is normal to wake up during the night. However, this is normally followed by falling right back to sleep. If your child is reliant upon your presence to fall asleep at the beginning of the night, then he will come looking for you if he awakens during the night.

Establishing a nighttime routine is the first step toward reducing sleep problems. Just as adults have nighttime rituals that are helpful to their falling asleep, so do children. A routine will not only signal to your child that it is time to go to sleep, but more important, the routine itself will also help to induce sleep. For example, many adults have learned that turning on the TV, reading a book or listening to music can bring on sleepiness.

Keep in mind that activities that occur before, as well as throughout the routine should be calming. That is, save rough housing for an activity that occurs earlier in the day. A typical nighttime routine would start with giving your child a bath, provided that baths are calming for him. Next, put on pajamas and brush teeth. If brushing teeth is distressing, then that should be done earlier in the evening. Reading a quiet story can be enjoyable as well as relaxing. This routine should occur every night and with no deviation until a consistent sleep habit is established.

SELECTING THE PROPER BEDTIME

When going to bed becomes an extreme control battle, it may be helpful to attempt to eliminate the conflict by increasing your child's tiredness. Establishing the proper bedtime may take awhile. In fact, it is advisable to start the routine at a much later hour than the time you would ideally like him to fall asleep. It is important that your child be tired, thereby reducing his resistance to going to bed. We have found it necessary to set initial bed times as late as midnight. Therefore, when parents announce that it is time to go to bed, the child is more willing. Gradually, the bedtime should be pushed up until your child is going to bed at the desired time. To help assist in your child becoming tired, it is often helpful to reduce or eliminate nap time. Not allowing your child to wake up too late in the morning is also advisable. Remember that the goal is that your child get the necessary hours of sleep on a reliable schedule.

DEVELOPING A "SLEEP" OBJECT

The most commonly reported sleep problem is awakening in the middle of the night. Although your child may still be tired, he does not know how to put himself back to sleep. This can be a problem for adults also, but typically adults think of something relaxing, turn on soft music or read for a bit. Since children do not know what to do, they often get up, turn on lights, listen to music, play with toys, wander around the house, or jump on the bed. They may seek company and climb into their parents' bed. Therefore, it is necessary to give them a means to put themselves back to sleep.

The best method is to establish an object or activity that is highly associated with sleep. Therefore, eventually being near the object can become an effective means of inducing sleep. For example, when your child is sleepy, give him a soft blanket. It may be helpful to stroke his face soothingly with the blanket. The blanket will eventually become associated with sleepiness. When your child wakes up, he will be able to use the blanket to go back to sleep. Use of stuffed animals or even a pacifier can also be effective. Eventually the pacifier can be eliminated. Playing soft music before bedtime can help develop a sleep association. Although there is concern regarding dental issues in giving a bottle to fall asleep, we have suggested placing a bottle in the crib to initially teach the child to soothe himself. Over time, water can be substituted for milk or juice. Once your child has learned how to fall back asleep during the night, he will eventually be able to do so without using objects.

Often children will wake up very early and not be tired. Rather than try to directly make them sleep, you should prevent all other non-sleep activities from occurring. There should not be toys available. Children should not have snacks or favorite beverages. The light should not be on. All cues in the environment should be suggestive of sleep, (i.e., quiet, dark, and still). You can provide a very low level of background stimulation if this helps, such as a night light and a softly humming fan.

STAYING IN BED

Undoubtedly, keeping a child in bed is the most difficult component of the program. It will require tremendous patience and absolutely no emotional reaction. The procedure involves continuously placing your child back in his own bed in a neutral manner. If your child gets up 100 times, you place him back in bed 100 times. Once he realizes he will always end up back in his bed and that he will receive absolutely no attention, he will give up.

If your child continuously gets out of bed, it will be necessary to place yourself near his bed or just outside the door to his room. To facilitate the likelihood that you will remain consistent, your positioning and comfort are important. Get a comfortable chair to sit in. Listening to music or books on tape through headphones will make the procedure more tolerable and may help keep your sanity. Once your child is sleeping in bed, you will fade your position to be farther away and out of your child's sight. Remember that this will take time!!! Changing sleep patterns is no easy task, but it will change through your patience and persistence. You will be rewarded with undisturbed sleep!!!

When placing your child back in bed, it is critical to use the least amount of physical contact necessary. For example, we would suggest that you use partial physical guidance rather than full physical guidance. Similarly, we would rather you use a gesture over partial guidance and a facial expression instead of a gesture. As discussed previously, there are multiple reasons for using the least directive method. First, it minimizes attention. Second, it reduces the potential control battle between you and your child. Third, it reduces a possible source of agitation. Finally, it is easier to fade. However, the foremost objective is to get the child back in bed in the shortest possible time with the least opportunity to fuss.

KEEPING CHILDREN OUT OF THEIR PARENTS' BED

Sleeping in one's own bed is an important part of being autonomous and independent, even for a child with autism. Unless you want him sleeping with you when he is an adolescent, you should not permit him to sleep in your bed now. By following the above procedure, having him end up in your bed is much less likely. However, if you find him sneaking into your bed it will be necessary to consistently place him back in his own bed. Once again, show no emotional reaction and use the least intrusive method necessary. As before, if he comes in your bed 1,000 times you must place him back 1,000 times. If the problem occurs frequently, you may consider using the above procedure.

If you permit your child to sleep in your bed, even infrequently, it will create tremendous difficulties. It is similar to winning a jackpot on a slot machine. One win is usually enough to keep people playing the slots hoping for that next win. Once in your bed may be enough to keep your child trying to get you to let him sleep with you for weeks. A second time might keep him trying for months.

Initially, we suggest that you do not make any exceptions. For example, if your child is sick or frightened, naturally you will provide comfort and care, but in his bed. If you permit him to come into your bed, he may not be able to make the distinction that he is sick and that illness is the reason why he is being allowed in your bed. And if your child can make the differentiation, he will most likely use the exceptions to test you unmercifully. Naturally, if it is age appropriate, he can come into your bed weekend mornings to snuggle and watch cartoons. Or you might set a time (e.g., when it is daylight) after which you will permit him to come in.

Sometimes parents wake up to the surprise of finding their child in their bed. The child has learned how to sneak in unobtrusively. If this is the case, place bells on your door so that when he enters the room it will be easier to detect his presence.

NAP TIMES

If your child still requires a nap, then it is critical that he nap in his own bed. This is to support the habit of sleeping in his bed. If he naps in your bed, on the couch, or on the floor, it is likely that cstablishing a nighttime routine will be far more difficult. As discussed previously, it may be advisable to reduce or eliminate naps so that your child will be more tired at night.

Toilet Training

Every parent cannot wait for the day that their child is out of diapers. Being toilet trained means no more messy diaper changes, no more lugging diapers wherever you go and no more clipping diaper coupons. Just as important, there are more opportunities for integration. Many children cannot attend certain programs because they are not toilet trained.

It is essential to wait until a child is ready for toilet training. Do not give in to the temptation to rush toilet training. Although it is possible to toilet train a 24-month old, it is usually not advisable. It can lead to major frustration for the child and parents alike. Many typically developing children will breeze through toilet training if you can simply be patient until they are ready. They prepare themselves through natural observation. With an autistic child, who does not learn well by observation, it is all the more important to wait until he is ready before you undertake toilet training.

READINESS

The average age for children without autism to be toilet trained is two years, six months. Consequently, one should not even consider toilet training until this age. The following factors should be considered before starting a toilet training program. First, the child needs to be not only chronologically age appropriate but also developmentally age appropriate. This means your child is able to withhold urine for 60 to 90 minutes at a time and can recognize the sensation of a full bladder. He should also show awareness around voiding. Typically, a child will look toward an adult before or after eliminating, or indicate that he has a wet or soiled diaper.

Second, compliance problems and tantrums must be minimal. The presence of behavior problems will seriously interfere with the process. The program entails the child staying seated on the toilet for at least 15 continuous minutes. Therefore, if it is unlikely that he will stay seated cooperatively, he is not ready yet. Additionally, his self-stimulation must not interfere with the ability to concentrate during the program. If he engages in continuous self-stimulation it is unlikely that he will be able to perceive the sensation of needing to go to the bathroom. Finally, if the goal is independent toileting, he must have the capability of locating the bathroom independently or communicating the need to toilet. Additionally, the ability to take off his clothes, wipe, flush, redress and wash his hands are also important.

THE EQUIPMENT!!!

We highly recommend that you do not purchase a potty chair. The goal is for your child to eliminate using any toilet. Therefore, the use of a special potty chair not only is unnecessary, it can actually impede accomplishing the objective of going in any bathroom. Save your money for the victory dinner after your child is toilet trained!!!

We do recommend, however, that you purchase an insert that is placed on the toilet seat. This will greatly increase your child's comfort and help make toilet training more successful. It is also often helpful to have a stool, so that he can safely and comfortably climb up on the toilet. The stool will also be important so that he can place his feet on it when he is sitting on the toilet. Typically, it is necessary to actually teach a child how to sit comfortably on the toilet. Placing his legs in an open "V" position so that he can be stable will enhance his comfort. For boys, it will also help ensure that urine goes in the toilet rather than on himself or on you. You can also get a deflector shield to use as part of the toilet seat insert.

Boys and girls should both start with sitting. This greatly eases bowel training as you are training for urine. After boys have been successfully toilet trained, they can be taught to stand when they urinate. This is often accomplished simply by watching their fathers or brothers. At that time, you will need to make sure they learn not to pull their pants all the way down in order to urinate. This will avoid embarrassment when they use a urinal in a public bathroom.

SCHEDULE TRAINING

Schedule training is the easiest way to begin toilet training and can serve as an alternative to intensive toilet training (see below). Although schedule training means that you are responsible for your child's toileting, it can be the first step in developing independence. However, being schedule trained is not the same thing as being trained for independent toileting. Schedule training is a very worthwhile step, but usually results in children being dependent on others to remember to send them to the toilet. It is often necessary to go on later and complete the training process in order to achieve fully independent toileting.

The goal of schedule training is to teach the child to void when he is placed on the toilet and to withhold voiding at other times. It is recommended that you start with taking the child to the bathroom every 90 minutes. On any occasion that he does not void, then the next interval should be shortened to 60 minutes. Once he voids then return to the 90 minute schedule.

A common mistake in schedule training is to take the child too frequently (e.g., every 30 minutes). Although he may never have an accident, he is less likely to learn to retain urine for the normal length of time. Remember that the objective of schedule training is for the child to learn to wait until taken to the toilet. Therefore, he gains control over bladder and bowel function, which prepares him for independent toilet training. Naturally, we would never interfere with him going independently and would create a circus of reinforcement if he did!!! **In fact, what often occurs is that a child will independently start going to the bathroom.**

Another mistake is only taking the child to the bathroom when he appears to need to go. This will promote dependence upon you and make him less likely to learn to go on his own. It also increases the likelihood of accidents occurring. As with most programs, consistency is critical. The child is counting on you to take him on a consistent schedule. If you make it random or when you think he has to go, it will greatly increase the time it takes for him to learn.

When it is time for the scheduled visit, take him to the bathroom and place him on the toilet. Every three minutes or so, reinforce him for good sitting. You can sing songs, look through books or he can play with toys. It is important, however, that he not be so involved in play that he cannot attend to the procedure. If he should void, provide a circus of reinforcement. Providing him special reinforcers that he can only earn during toileting will help make it a special event. Be sure, however, not to be so exuberant as to startle or scare him. Once he voids, he can get off the toilet and resume his normal schedule of activity. He would be returned to the toilet in 90 minutes. If he sat on the toilet for 15 minutes without voiding, then he should get up and return again in 60 minutes.

When a child has an accident, we use the following correction procedure. Have him help as much as possible with the cleanup. This should not be done punitively. It is just so that he can experience natural consequences and it should serve as a mild deterrent. A few children find the cleanup process reinforcing, in which case it should be omitted. Next, practice a few times going from the point of the accident to the toilet. Be sure to remain emotionally neutral. Do not be disappointed over accidents. Your child can learn as much from the accidents as he will from his successes. If your child is experiencing too many accidents, then you should adjust the schedule to make the intervals shorter between trips to the toilet. Once he is more successful, then you can increase the length of the intervals.

ONCE YOU START SCHEDULE TRAINING, DO NOT PUT YOUR CHILD IN DIAPERS OR PULL-UPS, OTHER THAN AT NIGHT AND DURING NAPS!!! Even when you are leaving home you should not place him in diapers. Otherwise you will create confusion and inconsistency which can seriously undermine the whole procedure. We understand this is quite inconvenient (having to change wet and dirty clothes, finding a bathroom, etc.) but it often means the difference between successful and unsuccessful toileting.

LENGTHENING THE SCHEDULE

When your child's accidents are occurring less than once a day, then start lengthening the schedule. Typically, we suggest adding 15-30 minutes. The goal is for your child to simply start going to the bathroom independently, which often occurs when the schedule is lengthened.

SHAPING INDEPENDENT TOILETING

Schedule training can be used as the bridge to the ultimate goal of independent toileting. Once your child has been successful with schedule training, you are ready to work toward independence.

The procedure is rather simple. Besides lengthening the schedule, instead of putting him on the toilet, place him on a chair next to the toilet. He should be unclothed. Continue to reinforce him about every three minutes for good sitting. Obviously, if he gets up and goes to the bathroom make it a circus!!! If he should have an accident, follow the accident procedure.

IT IS CRITICAL THAT YOU DO NOT PROMPT HIM TO GO TO THE BATH-ROOM!!! Even if he is wiggling and squiggling and showing every sign of having to go to the bathroom, resist the temptation to prompt him to the toilet. The reason is that he will become dependent upon you and it will delay his learning to go on his own. Try to be patient with the process. Remember that he can learn from having accidents, too.

Another word of caution--if the child starts to urinate while sitting on the chair, **DO NOT** instruct or prompt him to go in the toilet. Once again, he may become prompt dependent. Additionally, you will then be in a predicament of what consequences to provide. Do you reinforce him for using the toilet? That would also mean reinforcing him for having had an accident first. Do you have him clean up and practice toileting correctly? This would negate the partially correct use of the toilet. The answer is to let him finish the accident (you may want to duck or place a towel on his lap) and then follow the correction procedure. Whenever an accident occurs, repeat the previous step. Therefore, during the next scheduled training, place him back on the toilet instead of next to the chair.

With every success, move the chair farther from the toilet and add an article of clothing. For example, the second step would be placing the chair a few feet from the toilet and putting on underpants. Next, you would place him near the doorway of the bathroom with pants and underpants. Once he is far from the bathroom and fully dressed, this phase is completed. It would be helpful for you to conclude this phase by having him sit on a different chair or on the couch. This is to make it is as similar to everyday life as possible. As described previously, when he has an accident, (and he will!), repeat the previous step.

DRY PANTS CHECKS

During the final phase, you will no longer take your child to the bathroom. Now it is up to him to stay dry. Therefore, reinforcement for staying dry becomes very important. To ensure this, carry out dry pants checks on a regular basis. This consists of asking him if he is dry and having him feel his pants. At the beginning, the interval between checks should be every 15 minutes. If he has dry and clean pants, praise him warmly. You may also wish to provide a small tangible reinforcer, but the amount of reinforcement should be less than he gets for initiating going to the toilet and successfully voiding. When he has an accident, follow the correction procedure. Gradually, the checks should be lengthened (e.g., 30 minutes, one hour, three hours, etc.) and the intensity of reinforcement should become natural.

INTENSIVE INDEPENDENT TOILET TRAINING

Parents sometimes opt to start with intensive independent toilet training. As discussed previously, it is vital that your child have the prerequisite skills (i.e., developmentally ready, able to sit for a prolonged time, stays dry for 60-90 minutes, able to communicate his need to use the bathroom **OR** find a bathroom independently). Independent toilet training is similar to the procedure described in "shaping independent toileting," except it is done in a concentrated fashion. You can attempt to do independent toilet training in one day or spread it out over a few days. Parents often find it helpful to do it over a three-day weekend.

It is helpful to withhold your child's favorite liquids and reinforcers for a week prior to training. Therefore, he will be more willing to consume those liquids during the training, which will serve to increase the opportunities for voiding. Likewise, motivation will be higher if you have withheld his favorite reinforcers for a while.

Intensive independent toilet training can be separated into three distinct phases:

PHASE 1. The objective is for the child to understand that he is supposed to eliminate in the toilet. Place him directly on the toilet with no clothes on. Provide him with liquids and verbal reinforcement approximately every three minutes for "good sitting." When he voids on the toilet, **MAKE IT A CIRCUS!!!** After the circus, he can have a play break for about 10 minutes before returning back to the toilet.

He cannot have an accident during this phase, since he is on the toilet continually. This phase usually takes between 30 minutes and two hours before he understands that he is supposed to void in the toilet. Your indication that Phase 1 is complete is when he anticipates his voiding by looking for the urine to flow and smiling or becoming excited when he has voided (he knows the circus is coming).

PHASE 2. The objective is to develop independence. Follow the procedure described in the "Shaping Independence" section. As described before, place your child on a chair next to the toilet without any clothes on and wait patiently. Remember, **DO NOT PROMPT!!!** Follow the reinforcement procedures as well as the accident correction procedure. Let us remind you once again that accidents are an important part of the learning process. The procedure will undoubtedly involve a few successes followed by failures and back to success. As described previously, Phase 2 is completed when your child is fully dressed and far removed from the bathroom.

      PHASE 3. The purpose is to build generalization. As described before, you start by conducting dry pants checks frequently and then lengthen the checks.

TO PROMPT OR NOT TO PROMPT

      It has been mentioned repeatedly not to prompt going to the toilet. However, intervention is not black and white and there are always exceptions!!! Occasionally, during toilet training, it may be necessary to use prompts. If your child is not picking up the procedure, then you may attempt to use the least intrusive prompt (e.g., gestures, taking him close to the bathroom, a glance, etc.) to expedite his using the toilet. **IT IS ESSENTIAL TO RAPIDLY FADE ANY USE OF PROMPTS. OTHERWISE HE WILL BECOME DEPENDENT UPON THEM AND NOT LEARN TO TOILET INDEPENDENTLY.**

BOWEL MOVEMENT DIFFICULTIES

      It has been our experience recently, that children often successfully become urine trained but bowel training is more difficult. This may be due to many factors such as diet, reduced frequency of bowel movements, associated pain, or simply control battles. It is essential to arrange a medical exam is essential if bowel training difficulties are experienced in order to rule out any unknown medical problems.

In order to increase your child's motivation to have a bowel movement and reduce any possible power struggles, purchasing special reinforcers can be quite successful. Involving your child in the purchase of these items and making it a major event can be quite effective.

Place the reinforcers in a prominent spot and announce that when he has a bowel movement in the toilet (using the words he understands), he will receive the reinforcer. Save the big reinforcers for the first time he successfully has a bowel movement and for after he has a series of successes. Parents have often found wrapping reinforcers as a gift or making it a grab bag can enhance the excitement.

When your child has an accident be as neutral as possible, follow the accident correction procedure and casually remind him of how he will earn the reinforcers. Avoid at all costs making it seem as though you are angry or overly anxious for him to be successful. Otherwise you may feed into the power struggles or create one that does not exist.

DIAPER RITUALS

Children often develop rituals around having a bowel movement. This usually entails only voiding in a diaper and often in isolation (hiding in closets, behind furniture, outside, etc.). If this is occurring with your child, take comfort in the fact that you are not alone. To eliminate this ritual, it will take time and patience!!! Start by providing the diaper for him to only use in the bathroom. After he becomes accustomed to this new pattern have him help place the contents of the diaper into the toilet.

After your child is reliably using the diaper in the bathroom, you are ready to proceed to the next step. This involves giving him the diaper and having him sit on the toilet. Eventually, cut a hole in the diaper or fold it back so that he voids directly into the toilet. Gradually, cut or fold more of the diaper until it is no longer necessary.

NIGHTTIME TOILETING

We strongly suggest that you do not attempt nighttime toileting until your child is toilet trained during the day. Therefore, he should still be placed in diapers during the night or at naps. Nighttime toileting is quite different from day time. Whereas day time is considered voluntary, nighttime is reflexive or involuntary. When children do get up to go to the bathroom during the night, what occurs is that their bladder fills and the sensation of needing to urinate wakes them up. Some children sleep so soundly that they do not have this involuntary wake-up response.

The procedure is quite simple! Purchase a "Mower Bell and Pad Device." They can be obtained through specialty catalogues. The device sounds an alarm when only a few drops of urine fall on the pad. The alarm wakes up the child so that the association between full bladder and waking up is established. The alarm also has the effect of stopping the child from urinating further.

It is critical that you wake up with your child. This is to ensure that your child is fully awake so that the proper association is established between the sensation of a full bladder and waking up. Additionally, you may need to help him get into the bathroom as well as clean the pad. Once this routine is complete, he can go back to bed.

Occasionally the bell is not loud enough to wake up your child. Without waking up, he will not learn the reflex. This necessitates making the bell louder.

This procedure is successful in nearly all circumstances. On the rare occasion where it does not work, the problem may be insufficient motivation. This is evident when a child wets the bed in the morning rather than during the middle of the night. He is most likely choosing not to get up and go to the bathroom. If this is occurring, a motivational system similar to the one described in "Bowel Movement Difficulties" should be effective.

NAP TIME

If your child is not yet nighttime trained, then he cannot be expected to remain dry during naps. Therefore, he should be placed in diapers the same as during nighttime. Once he is nighttime trained, then diapers should no longer be used.

Eating Problems

Parents frequently report eating difficulties with their autistic children. Although parents typically are not as concerned with eating difficulties as with problems of sleeping or toileting, it is a significant issue. The most common problem is a self-imposed limit on the types of food eaten. Some autistic children may limit themselves to only three or four foods. The most obvious concern is for health risks and secondarily for the toilet training complications which can arise. Furthermore, behavior problems can occur when parents attempt to have their child eat a new food. Unwillingness to eat more varied types of foods can greatly inconvenience the family at home. Planning outings when the child will be away from home at meal time is more complicated. Going to friends' homes for dinner or out to restaurants can be frustrating experiences as well.

Eating problems occur for many reasons. While it is perfectly normal for children to have preferences for certain foods, autistic children can be far more insistent on eating only their favorite foods. Other children may resist only mildly, but autistic children with eating problems can escalate to tantrums and aggression if they are not quickly accommodated. Parents understandably may regard the eating problems as not important enough to engage in serious battle. There may be fear of malnutrition if a child retaliates by refusing to eat. Unfortunately, on a daily basis he receives reinforcement for picky eating as well as for acting out or threats of acting out. Over time he will become progressively more resistant.

Many parents have on occasion entered the battle over eating. Sometimes this works, but often the child becomes even more stubborn. He may go to the extreme of vomiting or refusing to eat altogether. There are children that would literally starve themselves. Once again, parents often find themselves in the position of having to surrender. Attempting to set limits and not following through actually makes the problem worse than just giving in.

As discussed with other behavior problems like toileting and compliance, we highly recommend that you do not take on eating problems until you are fully prepared to face the battle. Progress in this area will come more easily when you have made inroads in reducing other less challenging behaviors. You will already have established a track record of success for your child and yourself, and you will have more confidence and credibility.

FOOD SELECTION

As with most programs, we want to approach this problem in the most positive and proactive way possible. Therefore, our plan would not involve rapidly increasing the child's diet nor insisting right away that he eat foods we consider nutritious. Rather, the program begins with selecting a food that you feel the child would most likely accept. This may be a food that is similar in texture and taste to his preferred foods. For example, if he will only eat spaghetti, you may be more successful trying other types of pasta or noodles.

We have seen that some children find any variation in their favorite foods to be completely unacceptable. You would not dare offer a different brand of chicken nuggets!!! In such cases you might actually have more success with food that is very different from what he would normally eat. That way he will not be suspicious that you are trying to trick him. Trust is very important in overcoming resistance to foods. It will work best if you let him know clearly what you want him to do, but let him make the choice to do it. Although it is not our preference, often we have to start with junk foods or sweets. Remember the first goal is to increase the variety of foods a child eats as well as reduce the resistance to trying new foods. Also remember, **THIS IS A PROCESS!!!**

SELECTING THE TEACHING TIME

The introduction to new foods should occur under the most optimal conditions. Therefore, meal time usually would not be a good choice. No one feels like battling during meals. Additionally, it is probably a time that is already associated with the control battle and will only make your child more resistant.

You should select a time when your child is more likely to be compliant and you are not rushed. If you are both in a good mood, there is a greater chance that your child will cooperate and that you will have the patience to work through his resistance unemotionally. This may be after he has played, or when you come home from an outing, or when he simply appears to be in high spirits. It should also be a time when your child is hungry but not starving. This will increase the likelihood of his trying a new food, but not make him desperate.

If you can also select a time prior to a favorite activity, you can use the activity as a reinforcer when he tries a new food. Additionally, it will provide an incentive to quickly finish eating. Naturally, if he does not try the food, he will lose the opportunity to participate in the activity. It may even be helpful to establish a routine where he participates in a preferred activity at a certain time. Therefore, he would be more likely to understand the contingency and eat the food quickly.

INTRODUCING THE NEW FOOD

The program involves having your child try an extremely small amount of the new food. It may even be just a speck. Once he has tried this minuscule quantity, he can have a bite of his favorite food. In order to increase the reinforcement value of his favorite food, we recommend that he **ONLY** get to eat the preferred food when he has tried a new food. Therefore, in the selection of the favorite food, only choose those foods that you can and are willing to withhold at all other times. As mentioned previously, once he has completed the eating session, he can engage in a favorite activity. Gradually, the amount of the new food he is required to eat in order to get the reinforcer should be increased. You should be prepared to try many different foods and to keep trying a food in future sessions even if it has been refused.

If a child is extremely reluctant to eat a food, you can shape his behavior gradually. Start with looking at the food. Then move to picking it up and holding it near his mouth. This can be done as a nonverbal imitation exercise. You demonstrate the action and then say, "Do this." Cooperation should be reinforced with bites of the preferred food. Gradually increase the requirement in order to receive the reinforcer. Additional responses may include smelling the food, touching a finger to it and then licking the finger, or touching his tongue to the food. You can intersperse trials involving contact with the food with trials that involve simple and fun non-food related actions (e.g., clapping). This helps to maintain compliance and behavioral momentum. It also increases the time the child is in close proximity to the target food and the eating situation. Some children need to be slowly desensitized to the food including all the sensory aspects. They essentially need to experience the food as non-threatening. In time, with repeated exposure they will come to not only tolerate it, but actually like it.

OTHER EATING PROBLEMS

EATING AT THE TABLE. Many autistic children do not cooperate with parent preference that they stay at the table during mealtime. They prefer to wander around while eating, most likely because they find roaming more enjoyable than having to stay seated. Note that this is a different issue than getting them to actually eat the food that is offered. The point here is for them to learn that when it is mealtime, what the family does is sit together at the table. A child may choose not to eat, but still needs to remain at the table. Secondly, if he does eat at any time during the day, he should learn that we do it at one specific location, such as at the table. Eating should be regarded as an activity in its own right and should not be subsumed under other activities such as playing, walking around the house, or watching TV. It helps establish a discipline that will greatly reduce other behavior problems.

A good place to start is that all food remains at the table. If the child starts to get up to leave, he cannot take the food. This will keep him at the table as long as he wants the food. Do not be discouraged if this initially results in a tantrum. He needs to see that you mean what you say and intend to stick to the rule. The tantrums will subside when he realizes that he is not going to convince you to abandon the rule. Once your child has learned this first rule, it is time to impose the next one. That rule is: Once you get up from the table, meal time is over. There are no second chances and no snacks or food until next meal time. Although this may seem harsh, it will teach him to remain at the table. The final step would be remaining at the table for the sake of being with the family regardless of whether he wishes to eat. Initially, the time requirement should be fairly brief. You should arrange a specific signal to indicate that it is OK to leave the table. A very natural way to implement this would be that when his sister and brother are done, he may leave with them to go play.

EATING TOO QUICKLY. Slowing the eating pace can be accomplished through more formal Discrete Trial Teaching procedures. Treat every bite as a new trial and have your child place his utensil down at the end of the response. Reinforce him with praise (and anything else that fits the situation) and have him wait five seconds before the start of the new trial. Use differential feedback so that eating slowly as well as putting the utensil down receives the highest level of reinforcement. Prompt as necessary.

Play And Social Skills

Play and social skills are among the most important skills your child needs to learn. The quality of your child's life will improve dramatically through play and social connections. Deficiencies in these areas often lead to isolation, boredom and even depression. Being able to play with other children in a meaningful way will increase your child's happiness and provide him with a vehicle to learn important lessons about the world and how to get along with people as well as help abstract cognitive skills. As described below, there are many other benefits to teaching social and play skills.

FACILITATION OF LANGUAGE

Children's language development can be effectively stimulated through play and social skills. We usually see at least as much development of language through play and social skills as through structured therapy. Structured therapy is certainly an important part of the process but goes together with carefully engineered play and social activities to make a complete program.

Children are far more inclined to vocalize when they are relaxed and having fun. Speech and approximations of speech occur more readily on a swing, in the pool or jumping on a trampoline than when they are in a 1:1 teaching situation. Conducting overly structured discrete trials in a chair may actually inhibit language. Consequently, we suggest starting verbal imitation in a playful situation. It may be advisable to begin with Communication Temptations (please refer to "Curriculum") in unstructured environments.

Language is developed far more naturally through social interaction and play. Children learn from other children how to speak naturally and childlike. Adults teaching language to children often produce adult sounding language. For example, in response to the question, "How old are you?", children are sometimes taught to say, "four years old" or "I am four years old." Although this is a polite answer, it is far too formal and not how children typically respond. Three-year-olds do not even give a verbal answer; they simply hold up three fingers. Four-year-olds will hold up four fingers and say "four." Older children answer this question by simply giving the number (e.g., "five," "ten," etc.). Such non-child responses make the child sound unnatural and can sometimes complicate the integration process.

INCIDENTAL LEARNING

One of the fundamental obstacles in autism is the extreme difficulty children with the disorder have in learning through casual observation. Providing social and play opportunities as well as actively teaching skills in this area will greatly assist your child in learning how to acquire information through everyday casual experiences.

Whereas the majority of the information typically developing children learn is through observation and watching others, autistic children generally require direct teaching. Therefore, one of the most important goals of therapy is teaching children how to learn from others. Many programs are devoted to developing these specific skills, such as Joint Attention, group Nonverbal Imitation, and the Observational Learning Program.

Social and play interactions will become a primary forum for your child to learn a variety of skills and acquire vast knowledge. Naturally, for this to occur it will require careful and systematic intervention. However, the benefit will be that your child will learn in the most natural manner.

Autistic children often are more focused in structured conditions, thereby making teachers reluctant to work under less-structured conditions. However, if this is not addressed early on, the problem will only becomes worse and greatly impede the children's long term progress. It is essential that they become proficient at learning in less structured and more natural settings as soon as possible. It is through this process that successful integration is more likely to occur.

SOCIAL REINFORCEMENT

Perhaps one of the biggest benefits of social skills training is the importance that peers assume. Peers will become a significant influence for your child, often far more powerful than adults. We have often found that peers can stop inappropriate behavior faster, more effectively and far more naturally than teachers can. Additionally, their consequences are much less contrived. Adults tend to sound therapeutic (e.g., "Use your words," "You're not being a good friend," "Are you feeling angry?", etc.), while children will be far more direct, politically incorrect, natural and effective (e.g., "Don't do that!," "Give it to me!," "That's weird!," etc.). Their actions can also provide effective natural consequences such as taking a toy back.

With time your child will develop a desire to please his peers. This is a crucial hurdle in the intervention process. It exemplifies the process of internalizing the desire to learn. Peers will come to be natural supports for appropriate behaviors. Consequently, generalization is far more likely to occur. Adult monitoring subsequently becomes less necessary. We have found integration substantially more successful when peers are viewed as important by the autistic child.

RESISTANCE TO TEACHING SOCIAL AND PLAY SKILLS

If you are feeling resistant to the notion of devoting a great deal of teaching time and effort to play and social skills, you are not alone! The majority of parents do not view this as a priority and question the importance. These are comments we hear frequently:

"I am more concerned right now with getting him to speak"

"Once he has language then we can work on social skills"

"I don't want to take any time away from speech and academics"

"My other children don't have lots of friends so why should my autistic child?"

As discussed above, the answer to these objections is that play is an important avenue for enhancing language and learning in general. Additionally, although not all people are social, nearly everyone learns from observing social interactions. Therefore, it is essential that your child have an opportunity to learn this way as well! In terms of priority, we see play as paramount.

Another big reason why there may be so much resistance to working on play is that it is extremely difficult to teach these behaviors. Unlike language and academic skills, where you can develop a structured curriculum, teaching play and social skills requires far more flexibility.

The specific play and social skills you teach will largely be based upon the skills of the target group of peers. Therefore, we cannot give you a specific curriculum of play and social skills. For example, the toys with which peers commonly play will differ not only in regard to age and gender, but will also depend upon where you live. Naturally, play in India differs widely from play with in the United States. The toys with which children play in Boston can be quite different compared to Texas. Even neighboring areas of Long Beach differ in the types of toys and games with which children play. Therefore, we cannot provide a specific list or curriculum. However, the following are examples of toys and activities for different ages:

Ages	Toys/Equipment	Games	Social Interaction
2-3	See & Say Simple Puzzles Dolls Characters Shape Sorter Swings Cars Musical Videos Music	Peek-a-boo Interactive Songs Coloring Busy Ball	Solitary Play Ball Tea Party Chase Ring Around The Rosie
4-5	Lego Marble Maze Blocks Cars Puzzles Dolls Disney Figures Painting Play Kitchen	Candy Land Shoots & Ladders T-Ball Soccer	Tag Hide & Seek Play Dates
6-7	Computer Games Light Brite Crafts Stuffed Animals Action Figures	Uno Baseball Soccer Ballet Ice Skating Hockey Inline Skating Kickball	Sleep Overs Catch Dress-up/House/ School Build Forts Brownies/Cub Scouts Birthday Parties
8-10	Sports Cards Model Cars/Planes Barbie Pets	Street Hockey Baseball Basketball Tetherball 4-Square Rings/bars Gymnastics Video Games Lazer Tag Handball	Sleep Overs Sporting Events Catch/Pickle Girl/Boys Scouts Swim Parties
11-15	Roller Blades Music Books Make-up Jewelry Magazines	Baseball Football Tennis Water Sports Volley Ball Chess	Slumber Parties Phone Calls Dating Mall Movies with Friends

Similar to toy play, social behaviors differ just as widely as toy play. For example, how children initiate peer interaction varies widely. Whereas most adults teach children to approach and ask "do you want to play with me?", this in reality is not the way most normal interaction occurs. In some areas, children simply play next to a child and then gradually incorporate themselves into the play. Often children simply lead a new friend by the hand in order to facilitate social play. In some situations, children may simply make a comment as an initiation (e.g., "I have a toy like that") or ask a question (e.g., "where did you get that?"). No one way is better, there are just a variety of ways that children typically instigate social play. Thus, it is crucial to identify the way children play in your neighborhood.

Because of the tremendous variety of play and social behaviors, they are difficult skills to teach. Therefore, parents and teachers often fall back to the comfort of teaching more defined and structured skills. Although Discrete Trial Teaching techniques are used when teaching these skills, it requires far more creativity in its implementation. One must be subtler in prompting and providing consequences, for example. Additionally, it is extremely beneficial if the teacher possesses great play and social skills.

Perhaps one of the greatest sources of resistance is the feeling that the child's behaviors must be brought under control before play can be attempted. Behavior problems become much more evident in the less structured setting of play and social interaction. Naturally, this is not a good reason to avoid teaching these skills. In fact, it is just the reason to work on it. Additionally, it is essential to address behavior problems in all situations!!!

One final reason we have heard for postponing teaching these skills is the argument that children need language for social skills. Certainly language is helpful, but it is not essential. All one has to do is go to a park where children from different cultures are playing. You will quickly see that they are able to play beautifully even though they do not speak the same language. So go ahead and work hard on developing basic language and cognitive skills but do not delay getting started on play and socialization.

SELECTING PLAY SKILLS TO BE TAUGHT

In order to teach play skills, one must first decide what skills to teach. Careful consideration should be given to the selection process. Play Skills should include interactive ones such as board games as well as activities that are suitable for playing by oneself. Preference should be given to activities that are suitable for the child's age and gender and will facilitate joining in with peers.

AGE APPROPRIATE. One objective in teaching play is to give your child the skills that will lead to an increase in social play with peers. Therefore, it is essential to choose play that is typical for his age group. Although his abilities may not, as yet, be commensurate with his chronological age, we still suggest choosing toys that come as close as possible to his chronological age. In most circumstances, a child will be able to learn some level of age-appropriate skills regardless of his current developmental functioning. Playing with toys that are associated with a much younger age can have the effect of stigmatizing children and interfering with acceptance by peers. The selection of play items can also impact self-esteem and the maturity level to which the child aspires. Age-appropriateness also applies to other issues such as clothes, back packs, lunch boxes, haircuts, general appearance and interests. Appearance and level of play can subtly influence how adults view and interact with the child. You want to ensure that all teachers and caregivers have appropriately high expectations, giving him credit for being capable and mature.

The best way to determine age-appropriateness is to simply watch what toys other children are using. Naturally, a good method is asking children and their parents what their favorite toys are. You can also go to a toy store and ask or read on the toy what the recommended ages are.

GENDER APPROPRIATE. This can be a controversial topic since today's society is generally much more accepting of children playing with all different toys. While playing with dolls or in a toy kitchen used to be primarily thought of as "girls" toys or activities, many boys engage in such play today. Similarly, girls being involved in rough play and sports is quite common. Despite society's increased enlightenment regarding this topic, we still need to be cautious and aware of the toys and activities that are more likely to be used by your child's peers, so that integration is facilitated.

PEER APPROPRIATE. Although a toy or activity may be age and gender appropriate, that alone does not guarantee that it would be a toy that your child's peers typically play with. Peer appropriate means that a toy or play activity is likely to be accepted by the peers your child will be socializing with. In order to maximize the opportunity for integration, you should also look at what toys his peers are playing with. Otherwise, the probability of social play is greatly reduced.

YOUR CHILD'S PREFERENCES. Although you can provide external reinforcement for engaging in toy and social play, reinforcement will be most effective if it comes at least in part from the enjoyment your child derives from the activity itself. By exposing your child to various toys, you can determine the ones in which he shows interest. This may be demonstrated through facial expressions, vocalizations, or simply playing with the toy. It is also extremely helpful to assess which toys or activities provide the type of sensory input your child seems to prefer. A clue to this can be obtained from analyzing his self-stimulatory behaviors. For example, if his self-stimulation involves lights, motion or texture, look for play activities that include those components. Does he like sand or water? Try to make that part of the play. For a child that seeks visual stimulation, a marble maze may work well. Activities like cutting and pasting could be suitable for a child who engages in tactile self-stimulation. Sound making toys are usually good for those who engage in auditory self-stimulation.

Do not limit yourself to only those play activities that you think your child might enjoy. The purpose of this program is to expand the range of interests and that will take time to develop. Initially, it will be very important to provide huge amounts of reinforcement for engaging in an activity for even a brief duration. Be sure to keep the time requirement brief at the outset so that it does not become aversive. In time you will be able to increase the duration and gradually fade the rewards as the activities become intrinsically reinforcing.

Given the current array of possibilities, you can most likely find a toy that is age, gender, peer appropriate, and also incorporates your child's interest. Fortunately today, most toys provide a great deal of sensory input.

SOLITARY PLAY

Finally, you want whenever possible to select toys that can be played solo as well as cooperatively. One objective of toy play is that your child learn to occupy himself independently during unstructured time. Consequently, you should not limit yourself to games or toys that require two or more people.

TEACHING PLAY

Play skills can start out by being introduced in an informal manner. You should select three to five items to work on at a time. Some of the items can be incorporated into the more formal discrete trial teaching curriculum (e.g., nonverbal imitation program). Others are more appropriate to work on during play time. Gradually increase the length of time your child stays with an activity and increase the variety of responses your child makes with a toy.

It generally is advantageous to introduce play in an informal, "playful" manner, such as on the floor. However, it may be necessary to begin with a more structured teaching approach at the table. Besides reducing possible distractions, it may accelerate acquisition of play and better familiarize the child with the basic steps involved in a play activity. Instructional procedures will include demonstration, role playing and differential feedback. Once basic skills are learned in a more structured discrete trial approach, the child should continue to practice and develop skills in the most natural setting and most natural manner possible.

COMPONENTS OF EFFECTIVE TEACHING

Whether teaching a play, social, communication or self-help skill, you use similar teaching techniques. Effective teaching can be broken down into five parts:

1. Identify component steps (Task Analysis)
2. Teach one step at a time
3. Provide repeated practice
4. Use prompting and prompt fading as necessary
5. Reinforce successive approximations of desired response

Good teachers follow these steps whether teaching someone play or communication skills, or how to use a computer or to hit a golf ball. Teachers who are skillful use behavioral techniques whether they know it or not, from ski instructors to little league coaches to orchestra conductors to Sunday School teachers.

TASK ANALYSIS

All skills should be divided into teachable parts. This simplifies the skill and therefore reduces frustration. It will also help ensure that each individual step is understood. Additionally, it will promote consistency across teachers. It is **CRITICAL** that all staff use the same steps that are outlined in a task analysis, in the same order.

The easiest way to do a task analysis is to complete the skill yourself. Write down all the necessary steps. Then have someone else complete the task and note all the steps. Then compare task analyses and decide upon a single format.

The number of steps will be based upon your child's age and functioning level. In order to facilitate success, it is better to have too many steps than too few. Once you start teaching, it will become evident if you need to increase the number of steps or can safely combine steps. If your child is having difficulty, then you should break the task down further into additional steps. However, if he never makes a mistake, you should be able to consolidate steps, resulting in fewer components.

TEACHING ONE STEP AT A TIME UNTIL MASTERY

Often people want to rush through the teaching process. However, if you move on too quickly, it is likely that your child will not adequately learn the skill. Since each step is generally dependent on the previous step, the skill will eventually collapse. You must teach one step at a time!!! A new step will not be taught until the previous step has been mastered. You can consider a step mastered once the step is completed **independently** (i.e., no prompts of any kind are used) for three consecutive sessions with three different teachers.

You must decide whether you are going to use forward or backward chaining. Forward chaining starts with the first component. Once that is mastered, you proceed to the next, and so on. Backward chaining starts with the last step and then you proceed to the next-to-last step and so forth. Backward chaining seems to be less frequently used but is an excellent procedure. It allows the learner to continuously observe the correct performance of the task. Additionally, it provides higher reinforcement in the beginning stages because the learner gets to the final step more quickly. He experiences completing the task on his own even from the very first session. Having completed a task results in the greatest level of natural reinforcement.

CONCENTRATED TEACHING

In order to speed the learning process as well as enhance performance, it is important that your child receive multiple learning opportunities. All too often, teachers have a child perform a task one time and then move on. If it is a prompted response, then this does not provide enough opportunity to consolidate the learning. In the same way that a golfer would never go to the driving range and ask for one golf ball, a learner should never practice a skill one time. Your child must practice the skill repeatedly. By making the learning fun, varying the setting and/or materials whenever possible, providing prompting as necessary, and plenty of reinforcement, you can greatly reduce frustration and boredom that may be caused by repetition.

PROMPTING AND PROMPT FADING

Please refer to the section on Discrete Trial Teaching procedures for a comprehensive discussion on prompting.

REINFORCEMENT

Reinforcement was discussed in detail previously in the "Disruptive Behavior" section.

DEVELOPING INDEPENDENCE

One objective of teaching play skills is to have your child learn to play without monitoring and supervision. Initially, however, individualized instruction utilizing discrete trial teaching procedures will be necessary. Once your child has mastered the skill, it will be necessary to rapidly fade your monitoring. This needs to be accomplished in gradual steps.

Fading your presence usually starts as simply as not talking and not making eye contact with your child while he is engaged in play. Therefore, it is advisable to use verbal reinforcement only at the end of an activity. Because reinforcement will only occur at the end of the activity, the duration should initially be very short. Increase the duration only as your child is able to tolerate increased delay of reinforcement. Also, your presence should be slowly faded. Start with being next to him, then a few feet away, across the room, leaving the room for a second and then lengthening the time away from the room.

Play Stations can be extremely effective in developing independent play. Initially, you may set up a single station, where toys are placed. Later you can add a second station. Teach your child that once he finishes playing at one station, he should proceed to the next station. Eventually, the number of stations can be increased further. It will help if the toys have a distinct beginning and end to their play. Therefore, when he is done, it will serve as a signal to move to the next station. For open-ended activities, use a timer that the child can start himself.

Social Play

In preparation for the peer sessions, appropriate play skills should be identified and taught in 1:1 discrete trial sessions. When your child has learned a few play skills begin the peer interaction with brief sessions. For example, arrange for the peer to come over for 30 minutes. The first couple of sessions should be aimed at making the experience highly reinforcing for both your child and the peer. This may mean no formal teaching until both children are hooked on the experience through such fun activities as baking chocolate chip cookies, making Kool-Aid, playing with a great toy, and swimming in the pool. In particular, the peer should leave eagerly looking forward to the next visit.

These play dates provide the perfect opportunity to identify which play and social skills that your child must learn in formal therapy. Not only will you be able to identify your child's deficits but the peer's play, social and language skills will become the standard. Therapy should focus on developing the most critical skills so that further social dates will be productive and enjoyable.

Once the peer seems to be enjoying coming over to your house and your child has learned some of the necessary prerequisite skills, it will be time to start attempting to sneak in teaching. The teaching occurs during approximately three "trials" lasting no more than three minutes each. During each "trial" you do a different activity. Select activities that are interactive and enjoyable for both of the children. These "trials" should be invisible to the children. In particular, the peer should not be able to tell that you are doing "therapy." The adult's role should be as informal as possible. Do not overly structure the activity, but have in mind a script that you can fall back on if the play stalls or goes in a wrong direction. The script is really a guideline for the teacher to follow if prompting is necessary.

Each activity should be one that your child is already familiar with from previous training. For each activity you should develop specific goals for behaviors you want to occur. Examples include language to use, eye contact, turn taking, where to be, and what to do. Naturally, teachers should understand age appropriate language and behavior so that they can facilitate and promote interactions that will help the autistic child fit into the play of other children his age. Sometimes we adults view play with an adult eye and therefore create adult play behavior.

Be sure to reinforce the peer for cooperative behavior. If necessary, prompt the peer as subtly as possible to ask questions and give directives to your child. Make sure your child responds to the peer. Do not let the peer do things for your child. If your child takes a toy from the peer, facilitate giving it back. If the peer asks the adult a question instead of the child, have the peer ask the child. The adult should not become the focus of the peer's interactions. The goal is to be as unobtrusive as possible. **DO NOT INTERVENE OR INTERACT UNLESS ABSOLUTELY NECESSARY!!!**

Be flexible with the time guidelines. You may need to adjust them very quickly. Spontaneous behavior should always take precedence over the script. Never interrupt something positive that is happening. Do not be too quick to give directives or prompts so that there is ample opportunity for spontaneous behavior to occur.

Gradually lengthen the duration of the trials and the length of the overall play session. As both children become more familiar with the routine, you can introduce the concept of taking turns choosing an activity. It does not have to be an activity that both find highly enjoyable. Additionally, you should arrange play sessions with other peers so that your child learns to accommodate to the play styles of different children. In the beginning you should stick with one-on-one play dates. Later on you can organize play dates with two or more peers at the same time. Be aware that the interpersonal dynamics are much more complex in groups of three or more and this will present new challenges for your child.

EXAMPLES OF SOCIAL/PLAY ACTIVITIES

Teaching goals that can be accomplished within these activities: Labeling; Expanding Language; Describing; Requesting; Taking turns; Assisting each other.

Highly Structured - Indoors
Send windup car back and forth
Table games
Play catch
Build something cooperatively
Put puzzle together
Matchbox cars/train set/hot wheels/race set

Cooperative Tasks
Food preparation
Building

Creative Activities
Make something with Playdoh
Art projects
Construction

Outdoors
Ride on seesaw
Take turns going down slide
Roll ball down slide to other person
Take turns riding and pulling wagon
Sand box play

Language-based
Have peer be teacher for teaching program
Have your child be teacher for peer
Language programs: statement-statement; reciprocal questions
Conversation
Story time

Movement Games

Follow-the-leader
Ring-around-the-rosie
Hide and seek
Musical chairs; freeze dancing
Tag
Hunting for bugs
Cops and Robbers
Simon Says

Imaginative Play With Props

Act out scripts: "Thomas the train"; Aladdin
Build a "fort" or "tent"
Play with play sets: Lego; castles; doll house
Play "Doctor"
Dress-up
Pushing chair cubes around pretending to drive
Pretend store; shopping trip; ice cream parlor, etc.

SETTING UP PLAY DATES

Setting up play dates can be an extremely difficult chore, mainly because of the need to identify and recruit suitable peers. Because of your child's deficits in language, play and social skills, he may have not yet succeeded in making friends. Often, autistic children do not have the same social opportunities or as much exposure to activities that involve peers. So there is rarely a pool of ready and waiting prospective playmates.

Once your child exhibits a sufficiently low frequency of disruptive behaviors, it is time to expose him to situations where he can connect with peers. Obviously, if you begin this before the reduction of severe acting out behaviors, it is unlikely that peers will want to play with your child. Additionally, it may stigmatize your child and reduce the possibility for a future friend-ship.

You can start with taking him to the park, restaurants where children go (e.g., McDonald's, Discovery Zone, Chuck-E-Cheese, etc.) or activity centers. The advantage of starting with this type of activity is that you can leave quickly if necessary. These activities will give your child exposure to children as well as provide you the opportunity to begin teaching him the necessary skills. Often, you will meet other parents and begin to orchestrate friend-ships.

We find enrolling a child in group sports to be an excellent way to find peers. Soccer and T-ball have been especially successful. Team members typically go on group outings after games and practices as well as get together individually. Do not worry about your child being unable to compete or understand the rules. Most young children do not either!!! It will be necessary, however, to work on the skills during more formal therapy.

Perhaps the best forum to meet peers is at school. We strongly believe that school is vital for many reasons including that it is the typical learning environment and affords generalization opportunities. But the primary reason is for social exposure. You have a captive group of peers!!! It is a great place to identify prospective playmates.

Parents of typically developing children often set up play dates. Do not wait for some-one else to take the initiative. Younger children may first need to be exposed to play dates that have been orchestrated by their parents before they discover how much fun it can be and start requesting it on their own. Setting up a play date will require that you contact the parents and invite them to come to your house. It is often helpful to tell them that your child is really inter-ested in their child or that you and your child would really like to have their child over to play. We strongly recommend that you do not automatically volunteer talking about your child's diagnosis or the purpose of the visit. When you see that it is evident to the other parent that your child is different, you can casually mention that he is behind in his language and a little shy.

PEER SELECTION

Often you do not have the luxury of being highly selective. However, if you do have a choice, peers that have very good social, play and communication skills are preferred. Children without behavior problems are also preferred. A peer that is very popular is ideal. Popular peers often provide instant access and support for your child. But above all, you want a peer that will serve as an excellent model for your child. If the peer has behavior problems of his own, it will be very difficult for the children to learn from each other. It is not recommended that you try to do therapy with two children at once.

Typically, girls or boys older than your child are better for one-on-one social play. Not only will they typically have better skills, but they are usually more patient and will stay with your child. However, you have to be careful about gender. Check to see if it is cool to have a friend of the opposite sex. Finding a child who is a little parental can also be helpful. In larger groups it may work better to target children who are a bit younger, so that the level of play will be closer to what your child is able to do.

STAGES OF SOCIAL DEVELOPMENT

Just like with teaching any other skill, it is important to be aware of developmental levels when teaching social play. Also be aware that boys play differently than girls. For example, girls usually engage in more sustained play, whereas boys often do not stay with one activity or toy for very long. Additionally, girls tend to be more verbal and engage in more creative play. Boys' play is not quite as imaginative. Remember to avoid the pitfall of using **YOUR** conception of play. That will too often be in the adult realm.

The following are examples of stages of social development as described in the Brigance Inventory of Child Development. The age in years and months is in parentheses:

1. Engages in simple game with others, such as rolling ball back and forth (1-0)

2. Imitates actions of another child (1-6)

3. Watches other children play, and attempts to join briefly (2-0)

4. Plays alone, in presence of other children (2-0)

5. Watches others play and plays near them (2-6)

6. Plays simple group games (e.g., Ring Around the Rosie) (2-6)

7. Begins to play with other children with adult supervision (2-6)

8. Begins to take turns (3-0)

9. Takes turns with assistance (3-6)

10. Forms temporary attachment to one playmate (3-6)

11. Can usually play cooperatively, but may need assistance (3-6)

12. Takes turns and shares, without supervision (4-6)

13. Plays cooperatively with up to two children for at least 15 minutes (5-0)

14. Has several friends, but one special friend (5-0)

15. Plays cooperatively in large group games (5-6)

The Autism Partnership Curriculum for Discrete Trial Teaching with Autistic Children

John McEachin

Ron Leaf

Session Guidelines

Setting:
Initially, therapy should occur in an area of the house that is away from traffic and is closed off from the rest of the house. A bedroom or den is suitable. Distractions should be minimized until behavioral control is established. As the student progresses, make the setting as natural as possible. Deliberately allow distractions to occur. Move to different places in the house and outdoors for part of the therapy session.

Teaching Techniques:

DISCRETE TRIAL TEACHING

Discrete trial teaching is a specific teaching technique used to maximize learning. The technique involves: 1) breaking a skill into smaller parts; and then 2) teaching one sub-skill at a time. Each teaching session involves repeated trials, with each trial having a distinct beginning (*i.e.*, the instruction) and end (*i.e.*, feedback). Each part of the skill is mastered before more information is presented.

Prompting Techniques:
The least intrusive prompt that will facilitate the behavior should be used. Prompts range in intrusiveness from Physical Guidance to Demonstration, Verbal Cues, Pointing and Within Stimulus Prompts such as Proximity. In order to facilitate independence, all prompts must be faded as quickly as possible. Performance of a skill with less or no prompt should result in greater reinforcement.

Reinforcement Procedure:
Reinforcement is one of the most critical elements of therapy. The goal of therapy is that the student eventually perform tasks and behave appropriately under natural schedules of reinforcement (*i.e.*, occasional) and with natural types of reinforcers (*e.g.*, praise). However, it is often necessary at the beginning to provide tangible reinforcers (*e.g.*, food, drink, toys, interesting sensory objects and stimulation, music, etc.) and to give them frequently (*i.e.*, continuously). As the student progresses, the schedule of reinforcement needs to be thinned and more natural reinforcers utilized. This is accomplished by requiring two or more responses before earning a tangible reward, using a variety of reinforcers, and developing praise and smiles as meaningful rewards.

Staffing Ratio:

Initially, teaching will need to be done one to one. As the student develops good attending and listening skills, learns through observation, and is able to wait for his turn, then additional children can be introduced into the situation.

Mastery Criteria:

Mastery is determined when the student consistently responds correctly. Typically when successful performance occurs between approximately 80 and 90 percent over two to three days, mastery is achieved. Keep in mind that the criterion is arbitrary, and it is important to make adjustments depending on the student's learning pattern. Usually, 100 percent should not be used as the criterion since this can create frustration and lead to boredom. It is unrealistic to expect 100 percent performance since there will be mistakes due to a variety of factors other than lack of understanding.

Structure of Sessions:

The goal is to increase the session duration to two to three hours. Schedule as many sessions in a day as is productive for the student. For some children (*e.g.*, those who go to school part of the day), this may be one session per day. For many students, it will be two or three sessions per day. Allow breaks between sessions. The sessions will be more productive if they are spaced out through the day, rather than scheduled back-to-back. Similarly, the sessions should be evenly distributed throughout the week.

Each session should be balanced between work and play. Approximately 50 percent of the session time should be formally structured teaching programs covering areas of cognitive and language skills. Discrete trials should be conducted in series ranging from as few as three to as many as 50 or more, depending on the attention span of the student, need for reinforcement, and difficulty of the material. Between each series there should be a mini-break. During the mini-break, the student can be given a toy or other reinforcer to play with at the table, or may be allowed to leave the table to play. Often, leaving the table is the best form of reinforcement. The length of the mini-break should be proportionate to length of the work just completed. For example, if you did three quick trials and then let the student go, the break would be 30-60 seconds. If the teaching lasted three to five minutes, the break would be two to three minutes. If the teaching lasted ten minutes, the break would be about five minutes. These guidelines are approximate and should be adjusted to suit the learning pattern of the student. Note that although it might be possible to conduct longer sessions (*e.g.*, 20 minutes) early in the day, doing so often increases fatigue later in the day, and makes afternoon sessions less productive.

During the mini-break the therapist should record data, and prepare materials for the next series. However, it is important to monitor the student's behavior during this time and to reinforce appropriate play and absence of inappropriate behavior (*e.g.*, stim). Part of this time should be structured, with the therapist guiding the student to play appropriately. Part of it should be left completely to the student to choose an activity, without any demands being placed upon him (although the rules for appropriate behavior remain in effect).

The other 50 percent (not devoted to formal teaching of cognitive and language skills) includes the mini-breaks described above, structured play, and activities such as walks and going to the park. This allows for generalization of skills and extending behavior management to natural situations and environments. About once every hour there should be a longer (10-15 minute) break with a change of location, for example going outside to play. The change in setting and physical activity are important to maintaining the student's interest level and attention as well as providing a balance of work *vs.* play.

Making Sessions Fun & Natural:

1. Enthusiastic tones
2. Varied settings
3. Varied instructions
4. Interesting and preferred materials
5. Maintain high success rate
6. Sensitivity to child's preferences
7. Varied curriculum
8. Interspersing tasks
9. Varied reinforcers
10. Natural language

Discrete Trial Teaching

I. INTRODUCTION

A. Discrete trial teaching is a specific methodology used to maximize learning. It is a teaching process used to develop most skills, including cognitive, communication, play, social and self-help skills. Additionally it is strategy that can be used for all ages and populations.

The technique involves: 1) breaking a skill into smaller parts; 2) teaching one sub-skill at a time until mastery; 3) providing concentrated teaching; 4) providing prompting and prompt fading as necessary; and 5) using reinforcement procedures.

A teaching session involves many trials, with each trial having a distinct beginning and end, hence the name "discrete". Each part of the skill is mastered before more information is presented.

B. In discrete trial teaching, a very small unit of information is presented and the student's response is immediately sought. This contrasts with continuous trial or more traditional teaching methods which present large amounts of information with no clearly defined target response on the student's part.

C. Discrete trial teaching ensures that learning is an **active** process. We cannot rely on autistic children to simply absorb information through passive exposure.

EXAMPLE OF DISCRETE TRIALS: Teaching a receptive label

Antecedent ("A")	Behavior ("B")	Consequence ("C")
"touch juice"	touches juice; good attention	"great"
"touch cookie"	touches cookie; good attention	"terrific"
"touch juice"	touches juice; poor attention	"OK"
"touch cookie"	touches juice; good attention	"uh-uh"
"touch cookie"	no response; good attention	no reinforcement (student must understand what this consequence means)
"touch cookie"	no response; poor attention	"You're not looking"; "too slow"; etc.

II. COMPONENTS OF A DISCRETE TRIAL

A discrete trial has the following components: 1) Antecedent (instruction or other cue); 2) Prompt (this may not occur during many trials); 3) Student response; 4) Feedback or other consequence; 5) Intertrial interval. Each component will be described in detail below.

A. INSTRUCTION/DISCRIMINATIVE STIMULUS (SD)/SIGNAL FOR BEHAVIOR

1. The trial must have a distinct beginning. Often it is a verbal instruction, but it may also be another discrete event or a visual stimulus. The event that occurs at the start of the trial should signal to the student that the correct response will result in positive reinforcement. Such a signal is known technically as a Discriminative Stimulus (SD).

2. In the beginning stage of teaching or if the student is having difficulty with a certain skill, instructions should be simple and concise.

   a. This helps avoid confusion

   b. It also helps highlight the relevant stimulus or stimuli (e.g., "cookie" vs. "juice" instead of "touch the cookie please" or "can you show me which one is the juice?")

   AS THE STUDENT PROGRESSES, INSTRUCTIONS SHOULD BECOME MORE COMPLEX AND MAY BE MORE WORDY. USING MORE NATURAL LANGUAGE:

   - promotes generalization

   - prepares the student better to learn from incidental situations

   - makes the session more interesting

   ---

3. Make sure the SD (or instruction) is appropriate to the task. Think carefully about what it is that you want the student to do and then select a verbal instruction or other cue that is appropriate to link to the response.

For example, if you want the student to count, "One, two, three, four" the instruction should be, "Count". If you want the student to tell you how many objects there are, the instruction should be "How many?" and the student's response should be "Four".

4. Give the student **approximately** 3-5 seconds to respond. This provides an opportunity to process the information.

   However, the teacher must be sensitive to the pace of therapy that is optimal for the student.

   a. Too fast may result in confusion and chaos

   b. Too slow may result in inattention

   c. Gradually the pace should approach what occurs in the natural environment (often staff uses a rapid pace to maintain attention, therefore it is critical to eventually slow the pace)

5. The best learning occurs when the student is paying good attention. If the student exhibits poor attending, it is essential to focus on developing better attending skills. This is discussed in a later section.

B. STUDENT RESPONSE

1. Know in advance precisely what response and what level of quality you expect in order for the student to earn reinforcement. Use consistent criteria. For example, how close does the student need to come to touching his nose if the instruction was "Touch nose"? It should be obvious to any observer (and to the student!) what criterion is being used. Having a clearly defined criterion:

   a. promotes consistency among staff

   b. increases the likelihood of correct responding

   c. increases the objectivity of the teacher

   However, you should readjust criteria based upon the student's changing performance.

2. Beware of extraneous undesired behavior. If you reinforce when such behavior accompanies a correct response undesired behavior may also be strengthened.

   Example 1: The student gives you a good answer but is looking away. If you praise at that moment, you are likely to get more responses in the future with looking away.

   Example 2: You praise the student for touching her nose but by the time the toy reinforcer is received, she has fallen out of the chair. She may think the reinforcer is a result of falling on the floor.

3. Be sure to reinforce spontaneous desirable behavior such as making eye contact, good sitting, or spontaneous speech!

4. If there is no response within the time limit (3-5 seconds), treat inaction as a failed trial.

5. **SHAPE BEHAVIOR**: The goal is for the overall quality of responses to improve over time. This is done by gradually adjusting the requirement for earning reinforcement. (Differential reinforcement will be discussed further in the section on consequences.)

   a. Use differential consequences to simultaneously shape correct responding and appropriate attending behavior

      Example: Let the student take a break when fussing is decreasing rather than increasing.

   b. Use differential consequences to reinforce better approximations to desired target behavior.

6. Do not allow the student to anticipate the response. If the student starts responding before you finish the instruction then one of these things may be happening:

   a. You are being predictable. Vary the order of presentation so that the student cannot read the pattern.

   b. The student may be guessing. Do not allow guesses to occur, because the student may get lucky and make the correct response. Giving reinforcement at this time would only promote further guessing.

   c. The student may not be paying attention. Do not allow responses to occur when the student is not paying attention.

7.   Sometimes self-correction is an acceptable response and even highly valued. For
      example, if the student is attentive and corrects the mistake without any cues from the
      therapist you may want to provide reinforcement. The process the student is
      displaying (i.e., problem solving) is actually a very important skill.

      *However, it is important to repeat the trial at some point to make sure the response occurs without
      self-correction.*

C.   FEEDBACK/CONSEQUENCE

1.   The response should be followed immediately by feedback. Reinforcement provides
      feedback that the response was correct and increases the likelihood that the response will
      be repeated. Negative feedback and the absence of reinforcement provides information
      that the response was incorrect and decreases the likelihood of the response being re-
      peated.

      a.   CORRECT: Praise plus constantly rotating selection of backup rewards.

            Correct + good attention = best reinforcement
            Correct + poor attention = mild reinforcement

      b.   INCORRECT: Informational feedback that the response was incorrect.

            Incorrect + good attention = supportive feedback (e.g., "good try")

            Incorrect + poor attention = stronger corrective feedback (e.g., "no";
            "pay attention"; "you need to look"; "try harder"; "you can do it better"; etc.)

      c.   NO RESPONSE: After five seconds with no response, give feedback and end the
            trial. If attending and seat behavior is correct and no off-task behavior occurs, the
            consequence may simply be non-reinforcement. Be sure to insert an intertrial
            interval (see below). It may be necessary to clear the materials briefly to emphasize
            that the trial has ended.

      d.   OFF-TASK BEHAVIOR: If the student exhibits inappropriate behavior
            (e.g., getting out of the chair, grabbing, stimming, etc.) immediately give feed
            back, correct the behavior and end the trial. Do not wait to see what response
            the student gives.

2.   Feedback should be unambiguous in meaning. For example, do not smile while
      you are saying "no" or frown and say "good".

3. Consequences should be planned in advance and the criterion consistently applied.

   However, be sure to give spontaneous reinforcement for unexpected outstanding behavior and performance.

4. Reinforcement must be selected based on each individual student's preferences (e.g., not all students like lavish praise or food).

   Effectiveness must be monitored continuously and adjustments made as necessary.

5. The reinforcer must be faded as quickly as possible to natural levels of frequency, delays and intensity. At the beginning, the reinforcer may follow 100% of correct responses (continuous reinforcement schedule). As learning progresses the rate should be decreased to an intermittent level in order to:

   a. reduce dependency

   b. reduce external control

   c. approximate what the student will encounter in natural environments thereby promoting generalization

   d. avoid possible chaos (lavish reinforcers can often escalate the student's disruptive behaviors or may simply be overwhelming)

6. Use differential consequences. This provides more information regarding the desired response:

   a. Excellent response results in the best reinforcer

   b. Response which requires more prompting or is of lower quality gets moderate level of reinforcement

   c. Incorrect response, but good attention gets a mild informational "no" or "try again"

   d. Aggression or blatant off-task behaviors receive strong negative feedback

7. Use feedback that is informational. Examples are "keep your hands down", "you're not looking", "too slow", "say it better", etc. Informational feedback:

   a. provides more information

   b. is more natural

   c. models language

D.   INTERTRIAL INTERVAL

1.   Allow a few seconds to separate each trial. The pause will:

   a.   allow the student time to process the information (i.e. that the response made was correct or that the response needs to change)

   b.   allow staff time to process what just occurred (e.g. think about what reinforcement to use on the next trial, when to prompt, what step of the prompting hierarchy to use, how to word the instruction for the next trial, etc.)

   c.   teaches the student to wait, which will commonly occur in more natural settings

   d.   allows collection of data

   e.   makes the onset of the next trial more discrete

2.   You may need to remove or reposition stimuli to make the trials more discrete. Leaving the stimuli visible on the table between trials provides the student the opportunity to rehearse the correct response or may promote switching responses without paying attention to the instructions.

Although removing stimuli or looking away for a moment accentuates the discreteness of trials, it also provides a cue to the student to get ready. Over time, you will need to make sure that the student does not become dependent on these attentional cues by deliberately making the trials less discrete.

THE INTERTRIAL INTERVAL SHOULD BE ADJUSTED TO MAINTAIN AN OPTIMAL WORKING PACE

- Too rapid a pace may be chaotic and therefore result in poor performance and increase agitation

- Too slow a pace may create inattention

- Make sure the teacher is directing the pace, not the student

---

E. PROMPT

1. A prompt is assistance given by the teacher to promote correct responding. It should occur before the student makes his response in order to prevent an error from occurring. Generally, it is given at the same time or just after the instruction, but it may also occur in advance of the instruction. If the prompt is too late or ineffective and the student makes an error, the trial must be ended and a more effective prompt needs to be given on the next trial. Using prompts:

   a. speeds up the learning process

   b. reduces frustration

2. Consider the full range of prompt levels, including visual, position, pointing, full physical, partial physical, verbal, demonstration, matching for receptive, receptive for expressive, within-stimulus, recency/time delay, etc. These prompts can be organized into a hierarchy from least intrusive to most intrusive. Teachers should select a prompt that provides just enough assistance to ensure success, but never more than needed. Choosing the appropriate level of prompt:

   a. makes it easier to fade the prompt

   b. reduces prompt dependency

   Prompts should be used to avoid prolonged failure by providing necessary assistance. Try to maintain successful responding (approximately 80% correct responding is optimal for many students).

3. If the first prompt does not work, then move up the prompting hierarchy (i.e., increase the level of assistance). For example, move from a position prompt to a pointing prompt.

4. A frequently invoked "rule" is when two consecutive incorrect responses occur then a prompt should occur during the next trial. This rule was developed for situations involving a two-part discrimination and where students already had a basic understanding of the concept being taught.

   a. The first incorrect response allows the student to learn from the feedback. Therefore, the second trial would provide the student an opportunity to make the correct response.

   b. More than two incorrect responses indicates that the student is not learning from negative feedback. It may also exceed the student's tolerance for failure and the lack of reinforcement may lead to an escalation of negative behaviors.

IT IS ESSENTIAL TO BE FLEXIBLE WHEN DECIDING WHETHER TO PROMPT

- If the student has no understanding of the correct answer then you may prompt after one incorrect response OR even on the first trial

- If the student appears to understand the task after the second incorrect trial then you may give another unprompted opportunity

- If you have followed the "Wrong-Wrong-Prompt-Test" sequence and the test results in another error then you should move up to a Wrong-Prompt-Prompt-Test sequence. If the test still results in an error, then go to a Prompt-Prompt-Prompt-Test sequence, etc.

- Prompt whenever you need to help the student maintain a higher level of success

---

5.   If it was necessary to use a prompt, move quickly to the next trial and repeat the instruction with no prompt (or reduced prompt). Testing after a prompt is given:

a.   reduces prompt dependency

b.   provides the student an opportunity to demonstrate learning from the previous trial

   However, if the student is just learning the task or has had tremendous difficulty with the concept, it may be beneficial to continue providing the same level of prompt for several more trials

6.   If the student has made an error due to inattention or off-task behavior, then it is preferable to provide a consequence for the inappropriate behavior rather than give a prompt. Prompting at that point may only serve to reinforce the student for off-task behavior, since prompts make it easier to get the response correct. You should give corrective feedback regarding the off-task behavior and repeat the trial, still not prompting.

7.   Unprompted correct trials should receive the strongest reinforcement (e.g., praise accompanied by tangible backup reinforcer).

8.   Prompted trials should result in a lower level of reinforcement (e.g., mild praise such as "okay", "that's right", "yup", etc.). However, it is essential that at least some reinforcement occur on prompted trials in order to:

a.   Provide feedback that response was correct

b. Strengthen the correct response

c. Avoid pattern of failure

However, if the student requires an extended period of prompting, you should occasionally provide tangible reinforcers for prompted trials in order to:

a. Increase the student's motivation

b. Reduce the student's withdrawal and frustration

c. Provide an opportunity for the student to experience the more desirable reinforcer

9. Be hypersensitive to inadvertent prompts. Extraneous prompts result in the student not mastering the concept because of:

a. Prompts not getting faded

b. Inconsistent responding (i.e., performance will seem to be better with trainers who provide inadvertent prompts)

c. Heightened student vigilance to irrelevant cues

INADVERTENT PROMPTS			
Non-Verbal	**Patterns**	**Feedback**	**Other**
Glances Posturing Positional	Massed Trials Alternating What was not asked	Expressions Fast when correct Slow when incorrect	Mouthing Answer New object

10. Make a strong commitment to fading prompts. By using progressively less intrusive prompts you will promote greater independence and mastery of concepts.

11. One way of fading a prompt is to systematically increase the delay between the instruction and the prompt. This allows the student the opportunity to initiate the response before a prompt occurs. However, beware that if more than two or three seconds elapse before the prompt is given, any verbal instruction may not be retained in memory.

12. Whenever possible, use within-stimulus prompts (e.g., position). Within-stimulus prompts are easier to fade and direct the student's attention to the stimulus itself rather than some extraneous cue such as pointing.

III. ESTABLISHING ATTENTION

1. It is important to reinforce good attention when it occurs. Be sure your praise specifies what behavior has earned reinforcement (e.g. "That was GREAT looking!!!", "I love how you are paying attention", etc.).

2. For many students the best way to teach appropriate attending is to start the trial regardless of attending behavior. Let your student experience the natural consequence of not attending.

   This requires the use of highly motivating reinforcers.

3. The student will learn faster to attend to natural cues if the tasks being presented require close visual attention (e.g. finer nonverbal imitation responses, matching on finer details, chaining, etc.)

4. Another way to teach attending skills is to time instruction onset to coincide with spontaneous looking and/or pauses in off-task behavior. You can prompt by waiting up to five seconds before beginning a trial to see if the student spontaneously orients. Since the instruction represents an opportunity to earn reinforcement, the presentation of the instruction is itself a secondary reinforcer. For this to be effective it is essential that the task be motivating; otherwise the student will be happy to delay the onset of the trial. Additionally, waiting longer than about five seconds merely provides additional opportunity for the student to engage in undesired behavior.

5. If the inattention is extreme, interferes with learning and the above steps do not work, it may be necessary to give a specific cue (e.g. "look at me"). If the student does not understand the language, you can do a "look at me" program. Remember that this is a prompt which must be faded as quickly as possible.

AVOID EXCESSIVE CUING TO SECURE ATTENTION

Instructions such as "look at me," "hands quiet," "sit still," or calling the student's name, can easily become a habit that is very difficult to break. You should rely primarily on strong differential reinforcement for good performance and attending skills. This will reduce reliance on external cuing and help develop internal control.

For example, when the student spontaneously looks at the teacher, say "Hey, that was great looking!!!"

IV. GUIDELINES FOR MAXIMIZING PROGRESS

1. Conduct enough trials so that learning can take place.

   a. Session length should be gradually increased in duration to increase learning opportunities

   b. Do not exceed developmental age expectations for duration of attention span

   c. Do not conduct so many trials that the student becomes bored or frustrated

---

PROBLEMS WITH SHORT SESSIONS

- Reduces learning opportunities

- Breaks momentum

- Not natural, thereby reduces generalization and integration into school

- Short breaks may not be sufficiently reinforcing

---

2. If the student is having difficulty on certain tasks, arrange task order so that difficult tasks occur between easier tasks (i.e., "sandwich" the more difficult task—the "meat"—between the easier tasks)

    a. Easier tasks may increase the student's motivation

    b. Easier tasks may reinforce completion of more difficult tasks

    c. Builds momentum

3. End the session on a pattern of successes. This increases the likelihood that the student will want to return.

However, if the student is extremely frustrated it may be advisable to end the session anyway.

YOU DO NOT HAVE TO WIN EVERY BATTLE!!!

4. Create behavioral momentum. Response patterns established over a series of trials can facilitate desired responding over subsequent trials. To establish momentum, decrease the intertrial interval, prompt heavily, and spend only a very short time on delivery of reinforcement/feedback. Then give a bigger reinforcement at the end of a series of trials.

Another way to establish momentum is to create a pattern of success through "sandwiching".

    a. to increase compliance, switch to several trials of a high probability response. Higher probability responses include easier tasks, fully-mastered material, and ones that are inherently reinforcing.

    b. if there is a problem with echolalia or closure, embed the target response in a series of verbal trials that are not associated with the problem.

If a response is about to happen that you cannot control, insert an appropriate instruction, so that the student is actually being compliant (e.g., when the student is in the process of moving a block off the table, say "put the block on the floor").

5. When teaching a discrimination, do not promote "mindless" responding or mere perseveration on a response. If the student can get the next response correct without listening to the instruction, then you are not really teaching anything. Massed trials (repeatedly asking for the same item) can create this problem.

   Use expanded trials to force the student to concentrate on what you are saying. Insert a progressively longer series of distractor trials between trials on the target item.

6. Incorporate a good balance of play into the overall program. Play is critical in order for the student to have productive free time (*i.e.*, not engaged in self-stimulation). Play is also essential to help develop social skills. Most important, language is often facilitated through play skills.

7. BE FLEXIBLE & PATIENT; YOU CANNOT SOLVE EVERY PROBLEM TODAY!!! LEARNING IS A PROCESS. LANGUAGE, SOCIAL AND PLAY TYPICALLY DEVELOP THROUGH MONTHS AND YEARS OF INTERVENTION.

   However, it is not good enough for the student to respond only on his own terms. The adult must be willing to set limits and enforce contingencies.

8. Maximize contrast between positive and corrective feedback.

9. Do not confuse respondent behavior (frustration) with operant behavior (manipulation). If behavior is respondent, our approach will be much more supportive and accommodating, whereas with operant behavior we may need to be quite firm

10. Adjust training based upon the student's behaviors and performance!!! Progression is based upon the student's responses to the trials. From observing the therapist (e.g., complexity of instructions, level of prompting, schedule of reinforcement, etc.) one should be able to predict the student's current level of performance.

11. Keep long term goals in view. Everything you work on should be designed to move the student toward the long term goals. A program is not an end, but a means to the end.

12. MAKE TEACHING NATURAL AND FUN!!! While teaching needs to be systematic and some students may need a higher level of structure, it is not necessary to be overly regimented. Teaching should be as natural as possible to increase the student's motivation and participation and facilitate generalization.

MAKING THERAPY NATURAL, FUN & GENERALIZABLE

- Use enthusiastic tones

- Vary settings

- Vary instructions (e.g., "What is it?", "What do you see?", "Tell me about this?")

- Use interesting, preferred and functional materials

- Do not bore the student by continuing a program that is already mastered

- Do not punish the student for good attending and performance by dragging out tasks when the student is cooperative. Similarly, be careful about shortening programs when the student is fussing

- Maintain a high success rate

- Use the student's preferences (even self-stimulatory objects can be used as reinforcers)

- Intersperse tasks

- Use varied and natural reinforcers

- Use language that is as natural as possible

- Use a curriculum that is wide ranging in scope (e.g., language, play, social, self-help)

- Reduce structure as much as possible (e.g., sometimes work on the floor instead of in the chair)

13. Model natural language as much as possible without distracting the student.

    a. More like what student will encounter naturally

    b. Models more appropriate language

    c. Promotes better articulation

    d. Exposes the student to new learning

14. Develop spontaneity

   a. Reinforce spontaneous variations

   b. Fade prompts and cues

   c. Train expressiveness of communication

   d. Link behavior to naturally occurring antecedents

   e. In labeling programs, stress commenting instead of question answering.

   f. Use Communication Temptations; model desired language instead of asking "What do you want?"

15. Use observational learning, modeling and group instructions whenever possible.

   ONE-ON-ONE instruction should be considered as a prompt that needs to be faded!!!

16. Do not create over-dependence by hovering unnecessarily.

17. Use probes to test whether the student already knows material. If the student seems to know it, review quickly and move on to new material.

18. When repeating instructions, voice inflection reduces boredom as well as signals to the child that the teacher is aware that the question is being repeated.

19. Use a non directive approach as much as possible. Set the stage for desired behaviors and then provide reinforcement when they occur. B.F. Skinner called this "reinforcement control" as opposed to utilizing "instructional control". He postulated that reinforcement control was superior to instructional control, because it promotes generalization and internalization.

By reducing external control and using indirect means to promote desired behavior, the student is more likely to buy into the behavior and therefore offer less resistance. Additionally, approaches that reduce directiveness are easier to fade.

EXAMPLES OF INDIRECT INTERVENTION

- Instead of cuing the student to pay attention, reinforce attention when it does occur and, more important, arrange tasks to promote attention

- If a student is positioned on an extreme side of the chair present material on the opposite side

- If a student is echoing, teach him to say "I don't know"

- To reduce self-stimulation, teach the student alternative responses which are highly enjoyable and are physically incompatible with the self-stimulation

Generalization Checklist

As soon as Student has learned items presented in discrete trials, generalization steps should begin. If Student has previous experience, generalization can occur quickly. The main objective is to accomplish items 1 and 2 below (in any order) if it did not occur during the initial phase of training. It may not be necessary to specifically train every substep and you should be flexible in choosing the entry point or which substeps to work on formally. As long as Student accomplishes main goals 1 and 2, the skill can be considered generalized.

DATE
ACCOMPLISHED

1. Program completed with various sets of objects
    and pictures   _____

          _____   Program completed with objects (if applicable)
          _____   Program completed using objects in the natural environment
          _____   Program completed with photos (if applicable)
          _____   Program completed using pictures in books (if applicable)
          _____   Program completed using videos (if applicable)

2. Skill is utilized with family members, peers, and any other
    persons in natural settings with natural cues   _____

          _____   Program completed with different teachers
          _____   Program completed out of the chair
          _____   Program completed in various rooms
          _____   Program completed at school or other settings outside of the home
          _____   Program has been practiced with family members in a structured setting
          _____   Program has been practiced with peers
          _____   Program completed with natural language

Compliance

Objectives:

1. Teach Student to follow simple directives that may be accompanied by gestures to facilitate understanding. The goal is to promote willingness to comply with requests using simple language that he is able to understand

2. Items to be taught:
    Come here
    Sit in chair
    Hands still
    Bring me the . . .
    [other directives as needed . . .]

Procedure:

The compliance program is based upon facilitating Student's successful following of instructions by gradually increasing demands. Initially Student will only be asked to complete tasks that he finds highly preferred. For example, Student may be asked to eat a snack, play with a favorite toy, or even self-stimulate. Issuing such instructions is very likely to elicit compliance, thereby providing an opportunity to reinforce following instructions. Gradually the instructions will be a little less desirable while maintaining extensive reinforcement for compliance.

Phase 1:

Identify instructions that are typically issued at home. Determine the rate of compliance to the various instructions. Construct a hierarchy of instructions, ranging from those with the highest probability of compliance (e.g., "Eat the cookie.") to those with lower probability of compliance (e.g., "Give your brother his toy back.").

Phase 2:

The teacher issues requests with the highest probability of compliance. Reinforcement is provided upon compliance with these requests. When Student exhibits compliance for three consecutive sessions, move to Phase 3.

Phase 3:

The teacher issues the high probability requests established in Phase 2 along with a few requests with a lower probability of compliance. Reinforcement is provided upon compliance with the requests. When Student exhibits compliance to the new, more difficult requests for three consecutive sessions move to the next phase.

Phase 4:   Increasingly, requests to complete non-preferred tasks will be gradually introduced while requests to complete preferred tasks will be reduced.

Nonverbal Imitation

Objectives:

1. Student learns to imitate the actions of others

2. Imitation becomes the foundation upon which other important skills are based (*e.g.*, verbalization, play, social, self-help, etc.)

3. Imitation is the basis for modeling which is a very important type of prompting

4. Imitation facilitates a positive relationship between Student and teacher (*i.e.*, being like the teacher becomes reinforcing)

5. Imitation builds awareness of the environment

6. Imitation helps develop attending skills

7. Imitation is a simple task that can be used to establish or reestablish compliance and attention. It allows Student to easily earn reinforcement

Procedure:

The teacher demonstrates an action and says "do this." Student is to mirror the action of the teacher (*i.e.* if teacher uses right hand, he should use his left hand). The phases start with obvious large actions and progress to more subtle and refined movements. Imitations involving the manipulation of a physical object (dropping a block in a bucket) or produce discrete sensory feedback (ringing a bell) are generally easier to learn. Ones that involve moving body parts away from the body (*e.g.*, arms out to side) or a part of the body he cannot directly see (*e.g.*, nose, head) are more difficult.

As Student progresses, the verbal cue will be generalized to other phrases which have the same meaning as "Do this" (*e.g.*, "do what I'm doing", "copy me", etc.). As a final step, the action will be named (*e.g.*, "Clap hands"). This builds the knowledge base for following verbal directions. "Do this" is used at first to establish the concept of imitation, an essential skill that provides a nonlanguage-based means of teaching a variety of other skills.

Prompts:	Use physical guidance to move Student through the action. Gradually fade the prompt to a light touch and then a slight gesture.
Entry criter:	There are no prerequisites for this skill. It is one of the simplest skills we can teach. In-seat behavior and eye contact can usually be shaped at the same time this skill is being taught.
Mastery crit:	Student performs a response eight out of ten times correctly with no prompting. This should be repeated with at least one additional teacher.
Phase 1:	**Start with items that involve the manipulation of an object**. Teach each one individually in isolation. This means doing repeated trials of just that item with no other object in view. Once Student is successfully performing an action without prompting, then move in one or more distractor items on each trial. Also, each item needs to be used in more than one way in order to build attention and establish a discrimination. For example, some times you should drop the hammer in the bucket, instead of using it to pound the pegs in. Once two items are able to be rotated randomly, introduce a new item. As each one is mastered in isolation it should be randomized with all previously taught items.

Object Manipulation

Block in container	Ring bell (shake or tap)
Pop up toy	Stir spoon in bowl
Bang drum	Throw bean bag
Ring on cylinder	Comb/brush hair
Put on hat	Wave streamer
Shake tambourine	Pop-up toy
Tap table with block	Spin top (press down)
Stack block	Honk horn
Raise cup to mouth	Pull lever
Shake snow globe	Tap sticks
Roll car	Crash car
Put on sunglasses	Clap with blocks
Load/unload dump truck	Throw ball
Play piano	Rock doll
Answer phone	Blow whistle

Phase 2:	**Start when Student has mastered five items from Phase 1**. Choose three items from large motor list. As each one is mastered, add an additional item for training. Sitting down should not always be the response that follows standing up. For example, you can have Student clap his hands while standing.

Large Motor:

Raise arms	Arms out to side
Clap hands	Stamp feet
Touch nose	Wave bye-bye
Pat tummy	Touch mouth
Pat head	Slap knees
Cover ears with hands	Pull hair
Touch elbow	Touch eyes
Tap shoulders	Touch toes
Tab table with hand	Stand up

Phase 3: **Imitations away from chair**. Start when Student has learned five items from Phase 2. Teach responses that involve going to a location away from the chair, carrying out an action and returning to the chair. Student should remain in the chair until teacher has finished demonstrating the action and has returned to the chair.

Knock on door	Touch spot on wall with
March	extended hand
Drop marble down chute	Look out window
Mark on chalkboard	Put item on shelf
Put object in drawer	Open/close drawer
Turn on/off light	Throw item in trash
Roll car down ramp	Put doll to bed
Put shape in sorter	

Phase 4: **Imitates another person**. Teacher indicates someone for Student to imitate and says, "Do that."

Phase 5: **Once five large motor items are learned (Phase 2), add fine motor actions**.

Fine Motor:

Squeeze Playdoh	Roll Playdoh
Touch chin	Touch mouth
Touch eyes	Touch ears
Pick up penny &	Push button
drop in jar	Put small pegs in board
Make OK sign	Drumroll fingers on table
Make victory sign	Thumbs up
Pinch clothespin	Squeeze squeaky toy
Point	Spin top (with fingers)

This is an appropriate stage to begin oral-motor imitation. See the Verbal Imitation, Phase 2 (oral-motor imitation).

Phase 6:   **Continuous chain.** Once ten imitations are learned from Phase 2, have Student follow along with you as you link together a series of responses. Vary the responses to maintain interest and attention and promote generalization. Start with two or three responses and then continue on with longer chains. The goal is to give a single verbal cue and defer reinforcement until the chain is completed.

Phase 7:   **Advanced imitation.** Once ten imitations are learned from Phase 2 and five from Phase 5, go on to finer discriminations.

<u>**Discrimination Examples:**</u>
Raise one *vs.* two arms
Touch nose with one finger *vs.* whole hand
Wave bye-bye with right *vs.* left hand
Tap once *vs.* two times
Clap high *vs.* clap low

Phase 8:   **Two-step chains.** This requires the use of memory. Once 20 responses are mastered from any of Phases 1-7, begin chaining responses together into two-step responses (*e.g.*, put on hat and knock on door). Start with items taught in Phases 1 and 3. Demonstrate both responses while Student watches. If necessary, prompt him to wait until the second action is completed. Then have him perform the two responses. Once he is good at responses from Phases 1 and 3, begin using items trained in phases 2 and 5 (*e.g.*, clap hands and slap knees).

Phase 9:   **Crossing over** (*e.g.*, touch right leg with left hand; touch left shoulder with right hand)

Phase 10:   **Two responses at once** (*e.g.*, touch shoulder with right hand and knee with left hand; crossing arms)

Phase 11:   **Three-step chains.** Same as Phase 8, but Student performs three steps instead of two.

Phase 12:   **Imitates action in video.** Present visual stimulus and tell Student, "Do this."

a.   Single discrete action

b.   Two-step action (simultaneous)

c.   Three-step action (simultaneous)

d.   Continuous chain

e.   Two-step delayed

f.   Three-step delayed

g.   Freeze frame video

h.   Action in photo

Phase 13:   **Imitates action in pictures.** Present a picture of someone doing an action and say, "Do this."

Cross-refer: Imitation is incorporated into Block Imitation, Play and Verbal Imitation. It also will lead into Receptive Directions. Negation includes "don't do this." Please refer to those programs for more information.

Block and Construction Materials Imitation

Objectives:

1. Learn to use play object in an appropriate manner

2. Increase visual motor patterning skills

3. Increase attention and memory

4. Establish behavioral self-control (*e.g.*, not grabbing at blocks, throwing, etc.)

5. Increase fine motor skills

6. Teach looking at task materials and actions of teacher

7. Teach turn-taking

Procedure: This program can be done with any type of construction materials including blocks, Legos, Lincoln logs, or shapes cut out of colored paper. The teacher sits across the table from Student. Each person has their own pile of materials off to the side of the table. The teacher will create a structure using the teacher's blocks out in the middle of the table. Student will copy the design using his blocks on the table in front of him. He should copy it the same way one would copy a diagram. Use blocks that have various shapes and colors. Start with two or three blocks and gradually increase the number of blocks you are using.

Once structures are built, they should be incorporated into play (*e.g.*, driving a car under the bridge). Various types of blocks should be used such as Duplo or Bristle. Action figures and animals can be incorporated into the structure.

Prompts: Use physical guidance, demonstration, verbal prompts, pointing, or a combination. Gradually fade prompts so that Student is performing independently. As a prompt at the beginning, he should have only the blocks he needs. Later on, there should be additional blocks that will not be used in the construction.

	TOYS/EQUIPMENT	GAMES	SOCIAL INTERACTION
2-3	See & Say Stamps Stickers Simple Puzzles Dolls Characters Shape Sorter Swings Cars Books Music Videos Cooking Music	Peek-a-Boo Interactive Songs Coloring Busy Ball Marble Maze	Solitary Play Ball Tea Party Chase Ring Around The Rosie
4-5	Legos Marble Maze Blocks Cars Puzzles Dolls Disney Figures Painting Play Kitchen	Candy Land Shoots & Ladders T-Ball Soccer	Tag Hide & Seek Play Dates
6-7	Computer Games Lite Brite Crafts	Uno Baseball Soccer Ballet Ice Skating Hockey	Sleepovers Catch Dress-up/House Build Forts Brownies/Cub Scouts
8-10	Sports Cards Model Cars/Planes	Street Hockey Baseball Basketball Tetherball 4-Square Jacks Rings/bars Gymnastics	Sleepovers Sporting Events Catch/Pickle Girl/Boys Scouts
11-15	Roller Blades Music Books America Online Make-up Jewelry	Baseball Football Tennis Water Sports Volley Ball	Slumber Parties Phone Calls Dating Mall Movies with Friends

Entry criter: Student has completed three items from Nonverbal Imitation Phase 1.

Mastery crit: Student performs a response eight out of ten times correctly with no prompting. This should be repeated with at least one additional teacher.

Phase 1:   **Building a tower**. Provide blocks and say "build a tower." Start with a two-block tower and gradually increase the size of the tower. Four block towers are expected at an age of 1 yr.-6 mos.; six blocks at 2 yrs.-0 mos; eight blocks at 2 yrs.-6 mos.

Phase 2:   **Discriminates colored shapes**. Put out two different blocks spaced about ten inches apart (*e.g.*, a red square and a long green rectangle). Hand Student a block that matches one of the two and tell him to "put with same." This is to verify that he can discriminate between the blocks.

Phase 3:   **Sequential steps**. Put down a piece of paper to define the building area for each person. The teacher completes one step of the construction and waits for Student to copy the step. Proceed to the next step of construction. Record the number of steps completed and the number of prompts. Establish correct imitation of all possible placements, starting with the easiest and progressing to more difficult.

    a.   on top
    b.   left *vs.* right
    c.   front *vs.* back
    d.   orientation of block

Be sure to randomize the shape and color of the blocks used from trial to trial and also to vary the placement. The purpose is to establish generalized imitation, not to teach specific designs.

Phase 4:   **Prebuilt structure**. The teacher completes model structure before Student begins his structure. If necessary, this can be done behind a shield to ensure that he waits. Gradually increase complexity.

Phase 5:   **Copying block patterns with one inch colored cubes**

    a.   horizontal
    b.   vertical
    c.   combined horizontal and vertical
    d.   add front/back dimension

Phase 6:   **Copying block patterns with uniformly colored blocks** (*e.g.*, unfinished wood; large cardboard bricks).

Phase 7:   **Copying 2-D design** (photograph or drawing).

Phase 8:   **Creating specific structures**: table, chair, bridge, garage, car, plane, train, house, bed, sailboat, etc. Model an arrangement of blocks that looks like a specific item. Later a photo can be used, paired with a verbal instruction. Fade the photo and have Student build the item with a verbal instruction only. You can incorporate figures into the construction to make it clear what you have built (*e.g.*, lay a figure down on the bed). Incorporate play with the structures created (*e.g.*, drive "car"; put animals in corral; etc.)

Phase 9:   **Design from memory**. Show design for five seconds and then conceal it behind a shield. Student makes the structure from memory.

Motor Skills

Objectives:	1.	Increase large motor control: balance; strength; coordination
	2.	Increase awareness of body orientation in space
	3.	Increase fine motor control and visual motor coordination
	4.	Increase awareness of environment
	5.	Improve motor planning
	6.	Learn to follow sequential steps
	7.	Increase opportunities for social interaction
	8.	Establish new reinforcers
	9.	Expand play opportunities
	10.	Develop readiness for pre-academic skills
	11.	Develop readiness for self-help skills

Procedure: These skills can be taught in an informal manner. You should select three to five items to work on at a time. Some of the items can be incorporated into the Nonverbal Imitation program. Others are more appropriate to work on during playtime.

Prompts: Use physical guidance, demonstration, verbal prompts, or a combination. Gradually fade prompts so that Student is performing independently.

Entry criter: Student can sit in a chair, stand still, hold on to objects and pay attention to the teacher.

Mastery crit: Student performs a response eight out of ten times correctly with no prompting. This should be repeated with at least one additional teacher.

Gross Motor:

Stand/sit	Walk sideways	Bounce ball
Hop	Two-footed jump	Kick
Turn around	Run	Rhythm
Dance	Skip	Wheel toys
Somersault	Stand on one foot	Tricycle
Balance beam	Climb ladder	Bicycle
Walk backward	Play catch	Jump rope
Ice skating	Surfing	Bowling
Swing	Swim	T-ball
Shoot baskets	Gallop	Skiing
Throw bean bag	Volley with balloon	Skating

Fine Motor:

Turn doorknob	Cut with scissors
String beads	Sticker books
Fold paper	Roll clay
Puzzles	Pinch clothespins
Paper punch	Use ruler to draw line
Pouring	Shovel into pail
Pasting	Pegboard
Put object in/take out of container	
Draw with chalk on sidewalk	

Matching

Objectives:

1. Student learns to put together items that are associated

2. Increase attention to detail (*e.g.*, grouping boys with green shirts *vs.* boys with red shirts)

3. Develop symbolic representation (*e.g.*, picture represents object)

4. Learn how to use materials

5. Develop independence by giving Student multiple items to be sorted

6. Develop a skill that is often used in playing games

7. Establish foundation for development of receptive and expressive labeling

8. Develop a skill that can be used to introduce more advanced concepts (*e.g.*, same/different)

Procedure: Student sits at the table and the teacher sits next to or across from Student. Place two objects on the table, spaced well apart from each other. Hand Student an object that matches one of the items on the table and say, "Put with same." If the object does not easily lay on the table, it is helpful to use a plate or tray under each item. The target item must then be placed on the proper plate to be considered correct. Move the objects around after each trial. Eventually the number of distractors on the table can be increased.

To facilitate language as well as to utilize more natural language, once he has learned concept of "same," the verbal cue can be changed to phrases with the same meaning, including "match," "where does this go?" "find one like this," etc. Children quickly catch on to the strategy of matching and you will soon be able to omit the verbal cue entirely. However, when you are ready to move on to labeling, it is helpful to do matching trials where you name the object (*e.g.*, instead of saying, "Put with **same**," Teacher says, "Put with **cookie**"). This will let Student become familiar with the label.

To increase his motivation, utilize materials and concepts that would be of interest (*e.g.*, foods, toys, etc.).

Prompts: Use physical guidance, pointing or position prompt. Gradually fade the prompts until Student performs independently.

Entry criter: Student can sit in chair, and hold objects. If eye contact is poor, this is a good program to develop that skill since looking is essential to making the correct response.

Mastery crit: Student performs a response nine out of ten times correctly with no prompting with two choices, eight out of ten times with three or more choices. This should be repeated with at least one additional teacher.

Phase 1:   **Object-to-object (3-D).** Use identical pairs of objects which are familiar to Student including some that easily fit together (*e.g.*, bowls, cups, spoons, blocks, etc.). Select two items to start with. Put the first item on the table (do not put out any distractor). Hand matching item to Student and say, "Put with same." Gradually move in a second unknown item as a distractor on the table. When Student responds correctly approximately three times with distractor present and no prompt, repeat with item two. When item two is done, go back and review item one, then item two. Finally put out both target items at the same time and begin asking randomly for one or the other. This is called random rotation. As each item is mastered, select an additional item to train. Once the new item is learned in isolation, it must be randomized with previously learned items.

Nesting items:
cups	plates
bowls	baskets
upside down cones	pie tins

Once Student is good at matching at the table, this can be done where he moves around the room to find the matching item. You can hand him the sample item to take with him to make this easier. Later you can do this without giving him the item (he only looks at it).

Phase 2:   **Picture-to-picture (identical objects, persons, animals).** Start when Student has mastered 10 items in Phase 1. Use identical pairs of pictures. Select objects which are familiar to Student. Select two items to start with. Follow the discrimination training procedure described for Phase 1. As each item is mastered, select an additional item to train.

If Student has difficulty making the transition from 3-D objects to pictures, select a variety of items that are progressively flatter. Items such as

Tupperware lids, drink coasters, hot pads, or squares of fabric, can be used and the dimensions of thickness and texture gradually faded out.

Phase 3: **Picture-to-picture (identical pictures of action)**. Start when Student has mastered 10 items in Phase 2. Same as Phase 2, but uses pictures of action being portrayed.

Phase 4: **Color**. Start when Student has mastered 10 items in Phase 1. Use pairs of objects or cut out figures from construction paper which are identical in every respect except for color. The developmental age at which the skill is identified as emerging by the Brigance Inventory of Child Development is listed in parentheses by years and months.

    a.   red, blue (B: 2-0)
    b.   green, yellow, orange, purple (B: 2-6)
    c.   brown, black, pink, gray (B: 3-0)
    d.   white (B: 4-0)

Phase 5: **Shape**. Start when Student has mastered 10 items in Phase 1. Use pairs of objects or cut out figures from construction paper which are identical in every respect except for shape.

    a.   circle, square (B: 3-0)
    b.   triangle, rectangle (B: 4-0)
    c.   diamond (B: 5-6)

Phase 6: **Size**. Use pairs of objects or cut out figures from construction paper which are identical in every respect except for size.

Phase 7: **Object-to-picture (identical 3-D to 2-D)**. Start after Student has mastered 10 items in phase 3. Follow same procedure as Phase 2, except Student matches object to corresponding picture.

Phase 8: **Picture-to-object (identical 2-D to 3-D)**. Start after Student has mastered 10 items in Phase 3. Follow same procedure as Phase 2, except Student matches the picture to corresponding object.

Phase 9: **Find same (pointing)**. For this skill, Student is shown an object or picture, but the teacher continues to hold the item. The teacher instructs Student to "find same." The response is to point to the appropriate item. After this is mastered at the table, it should be done with Student finding items around the room.

Phase 10:   **Multiple dimensions (identical color/shape/size combinations).** Follow same procedure as Phases 2, 4, 5, and 6, except have Student match according to combined dimensions (*e.g.*, red circle *vs.* red square *vs.* green circle *vs.* green square). Hand him a red square and tell him to "put with same." The correct response is to put it with a red square. Putting it with another red thing or a different colored square would not be correct.

Phase 11:   **Sorting.** Start after Student has mastered ten items in Phases 1 and 2. Give Student two items at one time to sort, then gradually increase the number of items. The verbal cue is "sort." As a prompt you can say "Sort—Put with same." Extend to functional daily activities.

Sorting

Color	Groceries
Shape	Laundry
Size	Silverware, dishes
Pictures	Alphabetical
Categories	Clothing

Phase 12:   **Non- identical objects (3-D).** Start this when Student has mastered ten items in Phase 7 or 8. Make sets of items that are visually similar but not identical. An example would be different kinds of cookies. Have Student form piles of objects (*e.g.*, cookies *vs.* shoes). The verbal instruction is "Put with [cookie]."

Phase 13:   **Non-identical pictures (2-D).** Start this when Student has mastered ten items in Phase 10. Make sets of pictures that are visually similar but not identical. An example would be different dogs. Have Student form piles of pictures (*e.g.*, dogs *vs.* cars). The verbal instruction is "Put with [dog]."

Non-identical Matching:

cookies	cars	dogs	balls
shoes	shirts	flowers	books
people			

Phase 14:   **Non-identical object-to-picture and picture-to-object.**

Phase 15:   **Non-identical actions.** Match pictures of different people doing same actions.

Phase 16:   **Quantity.** Matches cards with same number of objects depicted (*e.g.*, three ducks with three stars)

Phase 17:   **Associations** (items that go together). Hand object or picture to Student and ask, "What does this go with?" He should put it with the associated item.

Associations

pencil/paper	shovel/pail
sock/shoe	spoon/bowl
pillow/bed	toothbrush/toothpaste
napkin/plate	coat/hat
swimsuit/towel	lunchbox/sandwich
chalk/chalkboard	scissors/paper
flowers/vase	tape/tape player
videocassette/VCR	shirt/pants
glove/hand	sock/foot
ball/bat	candles/birthday cake
paints/brush	bike/helmet
basketball/hoop	broom/dustpan
pitcher/cup	hairbrush/hair dryer
soap/washcloth	train/track
baby/bottle	crayon/coloring book
nut/bolt	hammer/nail
lawnmower/grass	vacuum/rug

Phase 18:   **Emotions**. Matches faces that depict the same emotion.

Phase 19:   **Prepositions**. Match pictures depicting different items in same locations.

Phase 20:   **Letters, numbers and words.**

Cross-Refer: Note that categorization is a more advanced concept than non-identical matching. Please refer to the categories program. Matching is also an early phase of reading and quantitative concepts.

Drawing

Objectives:

1.   Improve grapho-motor skills

2.   Expand leisure skill

3.   Expand imitation, social interaction, and creativity

4.   Learn to follow instructions

5.   Improve following sequential steps

6.   Increase readiness for school

7.   Increase readiness for stories

8.   Increase readiness for writing

Procedure: Student sits at the table and his teacher sits next to him. Use a marking pen, which is easy to hold, and plain paper or erasable board. The teacher demonstrates an action and says "do this," or uses other verbal directions as listed below. Always use left-to-right and top-to-bottom movement. Be consistent about how you have Student hold the marker and which hand he uses. However, do not attempt to force a tripod grip before he is developmentally ready. Organize your work on the paper in a systematic way. Do not jump all around the page.

Be playful in your approach. Besides drawing at the table, you can use Magna-Doodle, sidewalk chalk, wall murals or painting. You can make a circle into a cat face, lines into train tracks, etc. Generalize from marker to crayon, pencil, and so on, but most of the time, allow him to use his preferred medium. Look for ways to incorporate drawing into other activities (*e.g.*, draw boxes on sidewalk for hopscotch).

Prompts: Use physical guidance to move Student through the action. Gradually fade the prompt to a light touch.

Entry criter: Student can sit in chair, look at work, and hold pen.

Mastery crit: Student performs a response eight out of ten times correctly with no prompting. This should be repeated with at least one additional teacher.

Phase 1:   **Controlling pen/scribbling**. The teacher demonstrates action, says, "do this," and gives pen to Student. Any kind of mark on the paper is acceptable.

Phase 2:   **Discriminates pen movement: push/pull strokes *vs.* continuous circular motion**. The teacher demonstrates action, saying, "do this," and gives pen to Student.

Phase 3:   **Fill within outline (coloring)**. Start when Student can successfully perform Phases 1 and 2. Using one color, draw a simple outline such as a rectangle. Then have Student use different color to fill in the area. As a prompt, fill in an area about one-half inch wide just inside the border. As he gets better at staying inside the lines, decrease the width of the area that you fill in. Gradually increase complexity of figure and generalize to coloring books. Another way to prompt for this is to outline the drawing with white glue and let it dry. This creates an edge he can feel with the marker.

Phase 4:   **Painting**. Start when Student can successfully perform Phases 1 and 2. Begin with books that only require an application of water. The teacher provides materials and tells Student, "paint." Move on to using a paint set.

Phase 5:   **Tracing figures**. Start when Student can successfully perform Phases 1 and 2. The teacher makes a faint dashed line to make a line, circle or other figure. Student is guided to follow line.

Tracing Figures
Vertical line
Horizontal line
Circle
Diagonal
+
X
C (pointing in all 4 directions)

Note: Stencils can be use to prompt this step if necessary.

Phase 6:   **Connect dots**. Start when Student can successfully perform Phases 1 and 2. The teacher makes two large dots and tells Student, "connect dots." Progress from making simple lines to drawing figures such as a house.

Phase 7:   **Copying figures.** When Student can successfully perform Phase 5, begin imitation (copying) of the figures. The teacher draws figure and tells Student, "do this."

Phase 8:   **Copying drawings of familiar objects.** Start when Student can successfully perform Phase 7.

Face	House	Sun
Tree	Flower	Snowman
Car	Cat	Ladybug
Umbrella	Flag	Caterpillar

Phase 9:   **Draw shapes free hand.** Start when Student can successfully perform Phase 7, and Student knows names of figures to be drawn. The teacher tells Student, "draw [figure]." There is no visible model.

Draw figures:
Circle
Square
Triangle
Diamond

Phase 10:   **Uses ruler to draw lines.**

Phase 11:   **Drawing familiar objects freehand.** There is no visible model.

Play

Objectives:

1. Develop replacement behavior for self-stimulation

2. Develop skills that will allow increased independence and constructive use of free time

3. Generalize language and cognitive skills

4. Provide venue for development and use of imagination, creativity, and abstract thinking

5. Increase attention

6. Improve physical and emotional well-being and self-esteem

7. Provide opportunities for observational learning

8. Establish means for interacting socially with peers

9. Develop age appropriate interests

10. Improve quality of life

Procedure: These skills can be taught in an informal manner. You should select three to five items to work on at a time. Some of the items can be incorporated into the Nonverbal Imitation Program. Others are more appropriate to work on during playtime. These are also useful activities to intersperse between programs while Student is still seated in his chair. Demonstrate and/or explain how to play with toy. Gradually increase the length of time Student stays with activity and increase variety of responses Student makes with the toy.

Initially, Student will be taught prerequisite play skills in as natural a situation as possible. However, it may be necessary to begin in a more structured teaching environment. Besides reducing possible distractions, it may keep from stigmatizing him while he has not learned appropriate play behavior. Instructional procedures will include demonstration, role-playing and practice. Once critical skills are learned, he will practice and continue to develop skills in the most natural environment possible.

IT IS CRITICAL THAT PLAY SKILLS ARE AGE APPROPRIATE.
THEREFORE, IT IS ADVISABLE TO OBSERVE PEERS IN ORDER
TO IDENTIFY THEIR PLAY SKILLS. IT MAY ALSO BE
NECESSARY TO SELECT SKILLS THAT INCORPORATE
SELF-STIMULATORY BEHAVIORS.

Do not limit yourself only to those play activities that you think Student
might enjoy. The purpose of this program is to expand his range of interests and that will take time to develop. Initially it will be very important to
provide plenty of reinforcement for engaging in an activity for even a brief
duration. Be sure to keep the time requirement brief at the outset, so that
he does not find it aversive. In time, you will be able to increase the duration and gradually fade the reinforcement as the activities themselves
become intrinsically reinforcing.

Prompts: Use physical guidance, demonstration, verbal prompts, or a combination.
Gradually fade prompts so that Student is performing independently.

Entry criter: These skills should be started as soon as Student is making progress in
nonverbal imitation.

Mastery crit: Student performs a response eight out of ten times correctly with no
prompting. This should be repeated with at least one additional teacher.

GENERAL TEACHING STRATEGY

1.   Select target play skill.

2.   Divide the skill into teachable parts.

3.   Teach one step at a time.

4.   Make time requirement brief, then gradually expand.

5.   Provide abundant reinforcement, emphasizing animated affect ("WOW, isn't this
fun!!!").

6.   Fade the supervision while encouraging and reinforcing Student for appropriate play.

7.   If self-stimulatory behavior occurs at a high rate, look at the nature of the stim and
identify play activities that include that aspect. For example, use a marble maze for a
child that seeks visual stimulation; activities like cutting and pasting for tactile stim; and

sound making toys for auditory stim. Stim behaviors that interfere with the play activity should be redirected.

AREAS OF PLAY

These are examples of types of play activities that should be included as part of Student's play program:

1.   Sensory
2.   Toys
3.   Puzzles
4.   Arts & Crafts
5.   Media
6.   Board Games

DEVELOPMENTAL STAGES OF PLAY

The age (in years and months) at which these play skills typically emerge is given in parentheses. These norms are taken from the Brigance Inventory of Child Development.

1.   Engages in play that extends beyond self (*e.g.*, brushes doll's hair, rolls truck) (1 yr.-0 mos.)

2.   Simple pretend play (*e.g.*, eating, sleeping) (1 yr.-6 mos.)

3.   Imitates housework activity (*e.g.*, sweeping) (1 yr.-6 mos.)

4.   Associates object in play (*e.g.*, taking a dog for a walk (1 yr.-6 mos.)

5.   Uses toys to act out a scene (2 yrs.-6 mos.)

6.   Engages in domestic pretend play, for at least ten minutes (2 yrs.-6 mos.)

   ### Examples:

   1.   Pat-a-cake

2. Blocks:
   a. Pick up block
   b. Stacking
   c. Make horizontal row
   d. Designs, towers, bridges, buildings, etc.

3. Puzzles

4. Shape sorter

5. Legos

6. Doll: pat, hug, feed, rock, put to bed, etc.

7. Puppets: do pretend actions; talk back and forth; make puppets as a craft project; act out a favorite story

8. Truck: roll forward and backward, load and unload

9. Ball: throw, catch, bounce, kick, roll

10. Play objects: yo-yo; jack-in-the-box; bubbles; slinky; Playdoh factory

11. Rhythm and music activities

12. Singing and Dancing

13. Tea party; dress-up

14. Play sets: farm; gas station; airport; playland; doll house

15. Kits: Mr. Potato head; Erector Set Jr.; Brio trains; clock that disassembles

16. Table Games: Uno, Connect Four, card/match games, Old Maid, Go Fish, War, Jenga, dominoes, bingo, memory/Concentration, Sorry, Mastermind, Scrabble, Boggle, Don't Break the Ice, Ants in Your Pants, etc.

17. Movement Games: Red Light/Green Light; hide and seek; ring around the rosie; duck-duck-goose; tag; hot potato; red rover; follow the leader; Simon says

18. Sports: tennis; basketball; billiards; ping pong; T-ball; basketball; soccer

Songs

Objectives:

1. Expand Student's knowledge base

2. Develop potential reinforcers and potential calming stimuli

3. Stimulate language development

4. Develop additional means for interacting with others

5. Develop additional leisure activity.

6 Help make classroom integration successful

Procedure: Select songs of the type you think will appeal to Student. Be mindful of what is age appropriate. If he has enjoyed videos, music that is associated with favorite videos is a good starting point. Keep in mind that songs that are current favorites only got to be that way through repeated exposure. Songs that include movement are especially good for promoting interaction, anticipation, and language.

Examples:

1. Row, Row Your Boat
2. Wheels on the Bus
3. Old McDonald
4. Twinkle, Twinkle Little Star
5. Head, Shoulders, Knees, Toes
6. Itsy, Bitsy Spider
7. If You're Happy and You Know It. . .
8. Tigger Song (from Winnie the Pooh)
9. Hokie Pokie
10. Ring around the Rosie
11. This is the Way We [wash our hands, etc.]
12. Something in My Shoe (Raffi)
13. Knees Up Mother Brown (Raffi)
14. Shake You Sillies Out (Raffi)
15. Rock-a-bye Baby
16. Pat-a-cake
17. Where is Thumpkin?

18.   Four Little Monkeys Sitting on a Bed
19.   Open, Shut Them; Open Shut Them
20.   A-B-C Alphabet Song.

Independent Work And Play

Objectives:
1. Increase duration of on-task behavior

2. Develop independence

3. Promote appropriate leisure activity

4. Help make classroom integration successful

5. Decrease Self-Stimulatory behavior

Procedure: Child should first master the skill to be performed. The goal in this program is to increase the length of time child can remain on a task with no direction or feedback. It will be necessary to gradually fade the proximity of the adult.

Phase 1: **One activity**. Assign a task that Student is capable of completing in a short amount of time. Initially, tasks should be more preferred activities (*e.g.*, puzzles, looking at a book, games, etc.) and eventually should include chores (*e.g.*, hang up your coat, take out the trash, make the bed, clean up the toys). Fade your presence while **NOT PROVIDING ANY PROMPTS FOR TASK COMPLETION.** If Student completes the assignment within the allotted time, provide him with a preferred activity. If he is unsuccessful, have him repeat the assignment. Gradually increase the duration of the activity.

Play Examples:

Shape sorter
Puzzles
Blocks
Legos
Marble Run/Maze
Mr. Potato Head
Dolls/Puppets/Animals
Solitaire card game/Brain teasers (Rubik's cube)
Games
Drawing/Coloring/Painting by number
Cutting and pasting

Craft: make mask from paper bag; sand art; spin art; jewelry; weaving
Origami: plane; hat; boat
Building models: cars; planes; etc.
Filling in peg board
Looking at book
Looking at photo album
Playdoh, Slime
    -- sculpting
    -- forms or molds
Creepy Crawlers
Basketball, Handball, Tennis, Pitch Back, Jump Rope, Hula Hoop
Skateboarding, Bike riding, Trampoline
Brio trains
Hot Wheels
Lite Brite
Dot-to-dot drawing
Spirograph
Puzzle work books
    -- hidden pictures
    -- mazes
    -- back of cereal box games
    -- patterning exercises
Build a fort/castle
Dress up
Walk the dog
Dig for worms; hunt for bugs
Hand-held video games

Daily Living and Life Skills

Sorting (*e.g.*, socks, laundry, silverware, groceries)
Self-care tasks (*e.g.*, dressing, tooth brushing)
Painting nails
Gardening
Making lunch/simple food preparation/microwaving popcorn
Domestic chores
    -- pick up clothes
    -- put away toys
    -- clear table
    -- set table
    -- take out trash
    -- fold laundry
    -- make bed
    -- sweep
    -- vacuum
    -- dust

Phase 2:   Two activities in succession.

Phase 3:   Three activities in succession.

Play Scripts

Objectives:

1. Teach a greater range of play skills

2. Increase complexity of language

3. Increase imagination and creativity

4. Expand range of interests and increase topics for conversation

5. Provide opportunities for observational learning

6. Learn to follow rules, carry out roles and be introduced to community and societal norms for social behavior

7. Increase social interaction

Procedure: Scripts should be thought of as a prompt for the teacher on how to guide the play. Whenever Student is able to generate his own form of play, the teacher should depart from the script until the play stalls. Initially these scripts can be taught using nonverbal imitation or receptive instructions. In time, the goal is for him to generate his own variations on the play. The sequence of spontaneous play development is:

1. Scripts

2. Creative combination of elements from different scripts

3. Student invents new elements for a script

4. Student creates a new script for a designated topic

5. Student chooses a new topic and invents a script

Prompts: Use physical guidance, demonstration, verbal communication, pointing or position prompt. Gradually fade the prompts until Student performs independently.

Entry criter: Nonverbal imitation-continuous chain

Mastery crit: Student performs a response nine out of ten times correctly with no prompting with two choices, eight out of ten times with three or more choices. This should be repeated with at least one additional teacher.

Script 1:   Build items and create an outing. This is an extension of Block Imitation.

McDonald's Burger
Build the restaurant
Drive up to the menu
Order food
Decide on eating in or take out
Pay cashier
If eating in: Choose spot to sit; eat; clear tray; leave
If taking out: Decide where to go; eat; clean up

Other things to build: toy store; pet store; race track; clothing store; food store; pier.

Script 2:   **Going for a drive**
Build a street with blocks
Build a gas station
Drive to gas station
Park; pump gas; pay
Wash windows; check oil; fill tires
Go for a drive

Script 3:   **Treasure hunt**
Hide pieces of "treasure" (reinforcers) throughout the house. Try using parts of a Nintendo game or other favorite activity.
Make maps or write out clues on cards for the location of treasure. This is a great opportunity to use concepts like prepositions.
Along with each piece of treasure that he finds, there is a clue for the location of the next treasure. The treasure at the end is a big one.

Script 4:   **Three Pigs**
Build each house: straw; sticks; bricks
Role-play pigs and wolf: "I'll huff and puff and blow your house down."
Knock down house
Rebuild houses

Script 5: **<u>Pirates</u>**
Everybody sings "Yo-ho-ho"
Board ship
Fire cannons: load; ready; aim; fire; boom!
Sail to island
Find treasure map
Hunt for treasure

Script 6: **<u>Space Ships</u>**
Put on astronaut uniform, helmet, etc.
Buckle up
Blast off!!
Explore Mars, the Moon, etc.
Go on a space walk
Get caught in a meteor shower
Splash down in the ocean
Be in a parade

Script 7: **<u>Act Out a Story Book</u>**
Use a favorite storybook that has pictures on each page. Round up characters and props needed to act out the scene on each page. Examples: Just Grandma & Me; Mickey & Minnie Go To The Beach

Script 8: **<u>Pretend to Eat at Restaurant</u>**
Props: table, dishes, pretend menu, pretend food, pretend money
Drive up to restaurant; park; walk in
Be seated by hostess
Get menus and order food
Waiter brings food
Pretend to eat/drink
Waiter brings check
Pay and leave

Script 9: **<u>Beach Outing</u>**
Pack up car
Drive/park
Carry stuff; find spot on sand
Spread out blanket; put up umbrella
Put on sunscreen; put on sunglasses
Go out on boogie board
Build sandcastle
Look for seashells
Have a picnic lunch

Script 10:   <u>Farm set</u>
Build corral
Put in animals
Bring hay on tractor
Feed hay
Go for a ride on a horse
Get a drink of water

Other ideas: Scavenger hunt
Build a fort with pillows, blankets, and chairs
Magic Show
Do impressions of famous people
Juggling (pretend)
Castles
Act out "Toy Story"
Peter Pan & Captain Hook
Aladdin
Cowboys
Pretend grocery store, ice cream store, donut shop, etc.
Pretend camping trip; fishing; canoeing; etc.
Build pretend snowman and snow fort
Pretend trip to Disneyland
Act out going to the circus
Build a zoo
Build Splash Mountain
Pretend outing to a swimming pool (with little characters)

Cross-Refer: Independent Work and Play
Motor Skills
Pretend

Receptive Instructions

Objectives:

1.   Increase understanding of language

2.   Establish compliance

3.   Establish instructional control which can be used to decrease disruptive behavior

4.   Extend therapy from chair into the natural environment

5.   Develop attending and awareness (*e.g.*, in order for Student to retrieve objects when further away from teacher, he must remain focused)

6.   Increase duration of on-task behavior

7.   Increase memory

8.   Develop independence

Procedure: Initially select items that have been taught in Nonverbal Imitation. Instead of saying "do this," the teacher simply tells Student to perform an action. Start with actions that can be carried out while seated in the chair. Later, have Student move about the room, the house, etc. at progressively greater distances.

Gradually fade out the demonstration prompt so that Student is simply following the verbal direction. As he progresses, the complexity of the instructions should be increased and the distance between the teacher and Student should be increased. The teacher should become very unobtrusive in monitoring his performance.

As Student's attending skills improve, begin giving multiple step directions. Initially, tasks should be simple and generous time allotted for completion. Gradually increase complexity of the tasks while decreasing time allotted for completion.

Prompts: Use physical guidance or demonstration to move Student through the action. Gradually fade the prompts so that Student is performing independently.

Entry criter: Student can perform several actions in imitation.

Mastery crit: Student performs a response eight out of ten times correctly with no prompting. This should be repeated with at least one additional teacher.

Phase 1:   **Instruction with contextual cue**. Put a ball on the table and say, "give me ball." Move the chairs by a door and say, "open/close door." Put an object on the floor and say, "get [object]." Put out blocks and say, "Build blocks." When two responses have been mastered, have both contexts present and establish a discrimination.

Phase 2:   **Object manipulation**. These are two-word directions that link an action with a specific object. These responses may help facilitate recognition of the object in a different context, such as the Receptive Object Identification Program where the instruction is "**touch** object."

Verbal Direction-object manipulation

Roll car	Ring bell	Throw ball
Eat cookie	Comb hair	Put on hat
Use spoon	Kiss doll	Hug bear
Shake maraca	Answer phone	Fly airplane
Pat dog	Blow bubbles	Blow whistle

Phase 3:   **Carries out action presented in photo/drawing**. This phase is intended for students who have difficulty with the receptive language required in Phase 2. For students who are successful in completing Phase 2, you may elect to skip this phase or come back to it later. Show stimulus and say, "do this." This can be extended to a series of steps presented in a flip chart.

a. One-step sequence.

b. Two-step sequence.

c. Three-step sequence.

d. Extended sequences.

Phase 4:   **In chair**. Start when five items have been mastered in Phase 2. These are simple actions that can be completed while remaining in place.

Verbal Direction-in chair

Clap hands	Arms out	Smile
Stand/sit	Touch nose	Tickle
Wave bye-bye	Jump	Give me _____
Tap table	Eat _____	Take _____
Raise arms	Drink _____	Point to _____
Give me hug	Stamp feet	Blow kiss

Go/stop (drawing line on paper/rolling car)

Note: Children like to get a hug when they stand up. However, teachers should not let standing up always turn into an immediate hug, or Student will confuse the meaning of "stand up."

Phase 5:

Pretend Actions

Sleep	Drive	Airplane flying
Drink	Eat ice cream	Talk on phone

Phase 6:

Verbal Direction-out of chair, same room This can be started when five items are mastered in Phase 4.

Turn on light	Throw in trash	Knock on door
Close door	Run	March
Go/stop	Open door	Get tissue
Walk	Bring me _____	Put object on shelf

Phase 7:

Go to another room and return. Start this when Student has mastered five items from Phase 6. It is also necessary that he first learn the names of various places in the house. Example: Go to the kitchen.

Phase 8:

Go to another room, perform an action and return. Start this when Student has mastered five items from Phase 7. Example: Go to the kitchen and get a cup.

Phase 9:

Say *vs*. do. Student discriminates between directives for speaking *vs*. directives to repeat a phrase.

SD1: "Say, 'stand up'"
R1: Student repeats phrase.

SD2: "Stand up"
R2: Student performs action.

SD3: Random rotation of SD1 *vs*. SD2

Phase 10:   **Two-step instructions**. Once 20 items from any of Phases 2, 4, or 6 are mastered, you can also begin chaining responses together into a two-step response. It is easiest if you start with object manipulation responses using contextual cues, then fade the contexts. Later, move to body action responses. Only use actions that have previously been trained as one-step instructions. Tell Student to do first part of response, wait for Student to respond, then ask for second part of response. Gradually decrease delay of asking for second part of response, until you can say the entire direction all at once and Student can correctly respond. If prompting is needed to get to the second step, use a non-specific prompt such as "keep going."

Phase 11:   **Three-step instructions**. Once Student is performing Phase 10 at 90% accuracy, give him three-step instructions. Use same procedure as Phase 10.

Phase 12:   **Conditional directions**. This is an advanced skill. Teach Student to listen to a direction and decide if it applies to him. Be certain that he understands the concepts and can answer yes/no questions that apply to the concepts being used (*e.g.*, "Are you a boy?").

       <u>Conditional instructions:</u>
       If your name is John, raise your hand.
       All boys, go to your table.
       If you have shoes on, stomp your feet.
       If you are wearing blue pants, stand up.
       If you have a book, raise your hand.

Cross Refer: Many of the initial responses to be taught in this program should first be established in Nonverbal Imitation. Receptive Instructions leads into Task Completion and observational learning. There is also a section in Imagination that pertains to following verbal directions. The concept of "don't" (do something) is taught in the Negation Program.

Receptive Labels

Objectives:

    1.   Learn the name of objects, activities and concepts

    2.   Often the foundation of expressive labeling

    3.   Develop abstract reasoning (*e.g.*, making deductions)

    4.   Facilitate attending skills

Procedure:

Student sits at the table and the teacher sits next to or across from Student. Place two or more objects on the table, spaced well apart from each other. Tell Student, "touch [item]." Move the objects around after each trial. Many students will get more actively engaged in the task if the response is handing the item to the teacher. In this case, the instruction would be "give me [item]." As soon as possible, you should vary the instruction (*e.g.*, "Touch . . .", "Give me . . .", "Point to . . .", "Show me . . .", "Where is . . .?", etc.). Often, it is possible to omit the command word and simply name the desired item. This may make it easier for the student to zero in on the essential word. Interest can be increased by varying the way materials are presented. For example, Student could go around the room to find the named items or select the item from a Velcro board.

Select Objects That Are Motivating And Functional For Student To Learn.

Prompts:

Use physical guidance, pointing, or position prompt. Gradually fade prompts until Student is performing the task independently.

Entry criter:

Student can correctly match items (see Matching Program) to be trained or imitate action. Establishing some simple verbal directions can facilitate progress in this program but is not a prerequisite.

Mastery crit:

Student performs a response eight out of ten times correctly with no prompting. This should be repeated with at least one additional teacher.

Phase 1:

Requests. Use objects or pictures that represent items or activities that Student would like to access (*e.g.*, food, drink, play, television, radio, swinging, etc.). Ask Student, "what do you want?" When he points to the object or picture, his request is awarded.

Self-stimulatory objects should be included as a choice. The value of the self-stimulatory object will be diminished by Student choosing other objects (*e.g.*, cookie) over self-stimulatory objects.

Phase 2:   **Body Parts**. [Note: Phase 3 can be started at same time or prior to this step.] Start with one body part. Tell Student "touch your [item]." When the first item is performed correctly with no prompt for three consecutive trials, add a second item. Once the second item is performed correctly with no prompt for three consecutive trials, go back and review the first item. Keep reviewing the two items until Student is able to perform with randomized presentation. Add additional items one at a time and rotate with previously learned items. As each new item is mastered, add an additional item for training.

Developmental Stages
a.   Mouth, eyes, nose, feet (B: 1-6)
b.   Hair, tongue, head, ears, hands, legs, arms,   fingers, stomach, back, teeth, toes (B: 2-0)
c.   Chin, thumbs, knees, neck, fingernails
       (B: 3-0)
d.   Heel, ankle, jaw, chest (B: 4-0)
e.   Wrist, shoulder, hip, elbow (B: 5-0)
f.   Waist (B: 6-0)

Phase 3:   **Objects (3-D)**. This can be started at the same time as Phase 2. Use objects that are familiar to Student and have been previously trained in Matching-Phase 8. Select two items to start with. Put the first item on the table (do not put out any distractor), and say, "give me [object]." When Student responds correctly four out of five times with the distractor present and no prompt, repeat with item two. When item two is done, go back and review item one, then item two again. Finally, put out both items at the same time and begin doing randomized trials. As each item is mastered, select an additional item to train.

Labeling Objectives:
Clothing	Toys	Animals
Food	Household items	Furniture

Phase 4:   **Pictures of objects**. The teacher asks Student to point to the object in a picture.

Phase 5:   **Pictures of action**. The teacher shows pictures portraying various actions and asks Student to point to the named picture.

Phase 6:   **Pictures of people**. (Often, children can learn this as 2-D more readily than 3-D). The teacher shows pictures of persons and asks Student to point to the named person. Include self, family, staff, and peers.

Phase 7:   **People (3-D)**. The teacher asks Student to point to Teacher, himself, or another person present.

Phase 8:   **Retrieves two items.** (*e.g.*, "Give me cup and shoe")

Phase 9:   **Size** (big/little) (B: 2-0).

Phase 10:   **Color**. Be sure to make this as fun as possible. You must use objects that are alike in every respect except for color (*e.g.*, use colored cups and hide a treat under the color you will ask for). Use colored bulbs and when he is correct he gets to turn the lights on.

Developmental Stages
a.   Red, blue (B: 3-0)
b.   Green, yellow, orange, purple (B: 3-6)
c.   Brown, black, pink, gray (B: 4 0)
d.   White (B: 5-0)

Phase 11:   **Shape**

Developmental Stages
a.   Circle, square (B: 3-6)
b.   Triangle, rectangle (B: 4-6)
c.   Diamond (B: 6-0)

Phase 12:   **Color/object combination**

Phase 13:   **Two abstract attributes combined** (*e.g.*, size/shape).

Phase 14:   **Three attributes combined** (color/size/object or color/shape/size).

Phase 15:   **Pictures of places/rooms at home and in community**. The teacher puts pictures of places/rooms on table and asks Student to point to a certain one.

Phase 16:   **Emotions**

Phase 17:   **Quantitative concepts**

Developmental Stages
a.   Many/one; little/big (B: 2-0)
b.   Empty/full; light/heavy (B: 3-0)
c.   Short/tall; thin/fat; less/more; short/long (B: 3-6)
d.   Slow/fast; few/many; thin/thick (B: 4-0)
e.   Narrow/wide (B: 5-0)

Next Pgms: Attributes, categories, functions, community helpers, prepositions.

Functional Communication

Objectives:

1. Teach the power of communication through nonverbal modalities

2. Provide means of getting needs met for nonverbal children

3. Decrease disruptive behaviors caused by frustration at not being able to communicate

4. Provide foundation for the development of speech

Procedure: This program is used for students who are not ready to use speech to make requests. It allows them a nonverbal means of communicating with others. Use actual items or picture of items as a means for Student to express desire or need.

Prompts: Use verbal, pointing, or physical prompt. Gradually fade prompts.

Entry criter: Student can match identical objects.

Mastery crit: Student performs a response eight out of ten times correctly with no prompting. This should be repeated with at least one additional teacher.

Phase 1: **Choices**. Present two or more items to Student. Ask, "What do you want?" Give Student the item that he chooses and remove all other items. Wait awhile before offering choices again, so that there is a consequence for an incorrect choice. If Student gets frustrated because he is not getting the thing he wants, give him a prompt (point or hand-over-hand) to indicate the item you think he wants.

Phase 2: **a) Matching pictures to items**. Start this when Student has completed Phase 1. Put two or more items on table in front of him. Hand a picture to Student and tell him, "Put with same." Prompt as needed. Reinforce with a small amount of the item that is in the picture.

b) Matching items to pictures. Start this when Student has completed Phase 1. Put two or more pictures on table in front of him. Hand an item to Student and tell him, "put with same." Prompt as needed. Reinforce with a small amount of the item.

Phase 3:

a) **Pointing to picture of an object**. Put two or more pictures on table in front of Student. Show him an object (but hold onto the object and keep it beyond reach) and say, "Point to same."

b) **Pointing to object shown in picture**. Put two or more objects on table in front of Student. Show him a picture (but the teacher holds on to the picture and keeps it beyond reach) and say "point to same."

Phase 4:

Making a choice from a picture. Start this when Student has mastered at least five items from Phases 2 and 3. Leave a picture of a highly desirable item out within easy access to Student. Use a physical prompt to get him to pick up the picture of the desired item and hand it to you. Immediately name the picture and exchange the picture for the desired item. Whichever picture he touches, give the corresponding item to him. You should also use the pictures to represent activities around the house and outside. Go to the immediate area where the item/activity is located and conduct the trial there. Then have him immediately do the item represented in the picture (*e.g.*, eat food item, drink, go to bathroom, go to swing, etc.). Initially have Student be very close to the place where the item is located. Then have him hand the picture to the adult and immediately perform the activity.

Once he is responding consistently, you can increase the number of pictures presented. At first use a single non-preferred item as a distractor to ensure meaningful choices. Gradually increase the distance and number of pictures that are presented. Keep pictures available to Student as a means for him to express desires throughout the day.

Picture Communication (Sample Items)

Bathroom	Video tape	Walk outside
Music	Drink	Computer
Cheetos	Captain Crunch	
Ride in car	Swings	

Phase 5:

Following directions presented with a picture. Take pictures of Student carrying out various actions, such as those done in the Receptive Instructions program. Show the picture and tell Student, "Do this."

Cross-Refer:

Picture Exchange Communication System (PECS) by Bondy and Frost.

Communication Temptations

Objectives:

1.   Increase Student's desire to communicate

2.   Make communication fun

3.   Establish power of communication

4.   Increase spontaneous use of language

5.   Bring speech under control of appropriate environmental stimuli

Procedure:

This program is designed for children who have the ability to make reasonable approximations of simple words to express desires. Articulation need not be precise, but listeners need to be able to tell the difference between various words the child says. For children whose speech is not developed to this level, refer to the choice making programs and Functional Communication.

Arrange situations that will facilitate Student's need to make requests. This procedure was described by Wetherby & Prizant (1989). Some of the strategies listed below were previously described by Margery Rappoport in Maurice et al. (1996). If prompting becomes necessary, utilize nonverbal behaviors (*e.g.*, exaggerated leaning in or looking at him, shoulder shrugs to communicate a lack of understanding). As a last resort, a partial verbal prompt can be given, such as "I want . . ." Avoid asking direct questions such as "What do you want?" Do not ask him what he wants. Fade to even more naturalistic reactions such as pausing to allow Student to fill the void.

Prompts:

Start with full verbal prompt. Fade to partial verbal prompt then body language prompt.

Examples

1.   Eat a desired food or play with a preferred toy in front of Student without offering any to him.

Playdoh	Action figures
Train	Cookies

Give a small amount when the request is made to facilitate repeated requests.

2.   Offer a non-preferred food item or stick his hand in a carton of pudding (to elicit a verbal protest).

3.   Activate a wind-up toy; let it deactivate and hand it to him.

4.   Open a jar of bubbles, blow bubbles, then close the jar tightly and give the closed jar to Student.

5.   Tell Student he is all done working, but do not let him get up until he says, "I want to go."

6.   Initiate a social game (*e.g.*, tickles, tossing him up in air, etc.) with Student until he expresses pleasure, then stop the game and wait.

7.   Set up a game, leaving out one important part (*e.g.*, dice, spinner, game pieces, etc.), and say, "Let's play."

8.   Blow up a balloon and slowly deflate it. Hand the deflated balloon to him or hold the deflated balloon up to your mouth and wait.

9.   Start putting a puzzle together. After Student has put in a few pieces, offer him a piece that does not fit.

10.   Select an object Student desires or one that makes noise and place it in a container. Hold the container and wait.

11.   Set him up for painting with watercolors (*e.g.*, provide paper, paint, brushes, etc.) and give him a cup **without** water.

12.   Tell Student he can go outside and play but leave the door locked.

13.   When he gestures for a drink, hand him an empty cup.

14.   Serve dinner without a fork.

15.   Place him in the bathtub without any water.

16.   Hold a book you are looking at together upside down.

17.   Put a familiar toy together the wrong way (*e.g.*, put the arm in the location for Mr. Potato Head's hat).

18. Sing a favorite song and leave out a word and only continue the song if Student fills in the word.

19. If Student wants to be picked up, hold out arms but do not pick him up until he says "up" or an approximation.

20. Put him on a swing. Give him a few pushes. Then hold the swing, waiting for him to say "go" or "push" or a similar word.

Verbal Imitation

Objectives:

1. Building a foundation for spoken language

2. Increase vocalizations

3. Shape articulation

4. Eventually reduce echolalia (*e.g.*, by bringing speech under appropriate stimulus control)

5. Eventually reduce monotone and mechanical speech

Procedure:

This often works better if done in a less formal manner. Depending on the phase, there may not be an explicit direction given to Student. Often it works better not to use the word "say," but simply model the sound/word. It is very important to make this a fun activity and not to make it seem like a program. For some children, it may help to sit them in a chair. Some children do enjoy doing this as a drill, but many children will be more responsive if done in a play context. When modeling speech to Student, you will have to experiment to determine whether it works better to present visual material or not. Presenting visual material (*e.g.*, picture cards) gives a meaningful context to the speech, but for some children, adding the second modality is distracting. For those children who do not benefit from the simultaneous presentation of visual material, you can practice the physical skill of saying words separately from learning the meaning and later combine everything.

The teacher should be exceptionally reinforcing and if corrective feedback is to be given, it must be done in a very supportive manner. Be playful in your approach (*e.g.*, using tickles and saying things like, "Come on, you can say it!"). Be willing to give some non-contingent reinforcement to keep the overall experience extremely positive. Use a lower level reinforcer for sitting and attending behavior, saving the most powerful reinforcers for vocal production.

In order to facilitate language:

1. Select sounds and words that are more frequently emitted by Student.

2.   Select sounds that are developmentally appropriate (*e.g.*, "m" instead of "z").

3.   Select sounds that would be motivating and more functional (*e.g.*, sounds that animals make: "moo," "baah," "sss").

4.   Select words that would be motivating and functional for Student (*e.g.*, cookie, juice, TV, open, help, no, all gone, uh-oh, owee, whee, up, go, more, out, tickle, etc.).

5.   Show him a picture or an object during the task (unless this proves distracting).

6.   Words may be used while emphasizing a specific sound (*i.e.*, "**C**-ookie)

7.   Work in a fun situation (*e.g.*, at McDonald's, while swinging, in the sand box, at the pool, etc.).

8.   Imitate Student's sound.

9.   Signing or gestures may be useful as visual cues to be associated with vocalization.

Prompts: Use physical guidance or demonstration. Gradually fade the prompts until Student performs independently.

Entry criter: Student makes some spontaneous sounds and is developing appropriate eye contact and has mastered at least three nonverbal imitation responses.

Mastery crit: Student performs a response eight out of ten times correctly with no prompting. This should be repeated with at least one additional teacher.

Phase 1:   **Increase Vocalizations**. Any time Student makes a speech-like utterance, praise him. Work on this at times when Student is in a good mood and during times when he is engaged in preferred activities (*e.g.*, swinging, jumping, swimming, being tickled, eating, etc.). A good way to increase desired vocalizations is to repeat back to Student any sounds he makes. Note any activities that are associated with a higher rate of spontaneous vocalizations. Also use music, singing, and objects that move or make noise when Student uses his mouth (horn, whistle, bubbles, etc.).

Use songs with movement to elicit vocalization. Try to get Student to complete phrases that teacher starts. Try Twinkle-Twinkle Little Star, A-B-C's, Wheels on the Bus, Itsy-bitsy Spider, etc.

Phase 2:   **Oral-Motor Imitation**. Start this when Student has mastered Phases 2 and 4 of Nonverbal Imitation. Select no more than three items to start and add one item as each is mastered. The teacher demonstrates the action and says, "do this."

Oral-Motor Imitation

Touch tongue	Touch teeth
Blow kisses	Sing into tube
Roll head	Pucker lips
Blink eyes	Stick out tongue
Open mouth	Frown
Smack lips	Pout
Smile	Nod head yes
Shake head no	Bite lip
Puff up cheeks	Blow (match/hand)
Tongue in cheek	Tongue to corner of mouth
Wiggle nose	Wiggle ear
Flap lips (raspberries)	Click-click sound
Indian sound	Breathe in through nose
Suck in cheeks	Fish lips
Yawn	Cough

Phase 3:   **Object manipulation with sound**. The teacher says "do this" and demonstrates movement of an object and makes the sound associated with the object.

Roll car	"Vroom"
Slide rubber snake	"Sssss"
Play with lion	"Roar"
Play with kitty	"Meow"
Toy falls down	"Uh-oh"
Push train	"Choo choo"
McCauley Culkin (hands on cheeks)	"Oh no!"
Tickle with bee	"Bzzz"
Pick up phone	"Hello"
Bounce bunny	"Hop hop"
Send figurine down slide	"Whee"
Tickle with hands	"Tickle"
Hammer on hand	"Owee"
Push horn on toy car	"Beep beep"

Phase 4:   **Temporal Discrimination.** Start this once Student is frequently making a variety of speech-like utterances. Set up a fun situation for him, but still maintain a loose structure and try to keep him focused. Ask for sounds you have heard Student make. Tell him, "Talk." Prompt by modeling a sound you have heard him make on his own. Wait up to five seconds for a response. If Student makes <u>any</u> sound during that time, reinforce immediately. In this phase, it does not matter if the sound is the one you asked for, as long as it occurs within a couple of seconds after the request.

Phase 5:   **Imitating sounds and words.** Start this when Student is making temporal discrimination (Phase 4) 80 percent of the time. Start with five easy sounds or words and add additional ones as each is mastered. If he is echolalic or says words spontaneously, you may also ask for those words you have heard him say. Also, pick sounds that are part of words that are functional for him. This includes favorite foods or toys and everyday items that are familiar (*e.g.*, shoe). Tell Student, "Say, '[sound/word].'" Emphasize the sound or part of the word that he can most readily say. It may be helpful to show the item as you are saying the word, but this can be distracting for some children. The following sounds are listed in order of increasing developmental age.

Easy Vowels
ah; oh; oo (boot); ee; ay

Easy Consonants
m; b; p; d

More Difficult Sounds
w, h, t, n
aw, uh, oo (book), er, ar
a (cat), e (get), i (hit), eye, you, ow, oy
g, k, f, v, ng, y
r, l, ch, sh, th (that), zh
s, z, j, th (thin), wh

Phase 6:   **Blends.** Start this when Student has mastered at least five sounds from Phase 5. Use syllables consisting of consonant and vowel sounds Student has already learned. Tell Student to make first part of syllable, wait for him to respond, then ask for the second part of the syllable. Gradually decrease delay of asking for the second part of the syllable until you can say the entire syllable all at once and Student can correctly respond.

Blends
M + ah, oh, oo, ee, ay
B + _____

D + _____
uh, ay, oo, + P
uh, ay, eye, + S

Phase 7: **Sounds without visual cues**. Start this when Student has mastered at least 10 sounds from Phase 5. Tell him to make sound/word, but cover your mouth so that he cannot see how you make the sound.

Phase 8: **Imitate Modulation**. Ask Student to say a word or sound. Only reinforce responses which match the way you made the sound.

Modulation
Loud/Soft	Inflection
Pitch	Long/Short

Phase 9: **Chains**. Have Student combine single syllables into two syllable words.

Homogeneous: mama; bye-bye; poo-poo; etc.
One vs. two syllable discriminations: da vs. dada; boo vs. booboo; etc.
Heterogeneous: mom-mee; coo-kie; ba-by; etc.

Phase 10: **Word Imitation/articulation**. Have Student imitate words and use shaping to get better articulation. Target sounds that are age-appropriate and that he sometimes says correctly, but has not yet mastered. Particularly important are articulation errors that reduce his intelligibility. Use lavish praise and prized backup reinforcers for better approximations of desired sounds. Intermix sounds that he can say better, to maintain confidence. Be careful not to overdo correcting his speech. You should accept the better 75 to 90 percent of his production. For production that is of intermediate quality, you can praise him and model better speech, but not ask for him to repeat it. Only the worst 10 to 25 percent of his articulation should be targeted for correction. An example of corrective feedback is "Say it like this, 'C-O-O-K-I-E.'"

To make practicing of verbal imitation more interesting, you can incorporate this drill into another activity. For example, with children who like puzzles or block building, you can have them say a word and then they receive the puzzle piece or block to put together. Try this with picture cards, with the reinforcer for saying the word being the opportunity to hold and look at the picture. Imitation can be done as you are looking at a picture book together. You can also do this while you are playing catch with a ball, jumping on a trampoline, swimming, sliding, etc.

Phase 11: **Imitating Phrases**. Have Student imitate two to five word phrases with clear articulation. It is common that the quality of articulation decreases as the length of the sentence increases. You should practice at the length that is just slightly more than what Student can easily imitate. If that is around three words, break longer sentences into clusters of two to three words. Try to group words together into natural phrases so Student's speech does not sound choppy.

ARTICULATION DIFFICULTIES

Many young autistic children with whom you will be working are just learning to speak. Keep in mind the child's developmental level. When we are interacting with a neurotypical 12-month old, we instinctively know not to correct articulation errors, but rather are thrilled with any attempts the child makes to communicate verbally. We should do the same thing with a three- or four-year old autistic child whose speech is at the 12 month level, namely model back the word articulated clearly. Besides learning, speech is a developmental process that should be given reasonable time to unfold. When there is a lack of progress, then the following strategies can help:

1.   When working on verbal imitation it is critical to make the experience as positive as possible.

2.   If corrective feedback is to be used **AT ALL**, it should be done in a supportive manner.

3.   When sounds are not articulated clearly, initially accept and reinforce response.

4.   When Student is learning to speak, shape articulation (*i.e.*, slowly require better approximations).

5.   Initially, accept Student's poor pronunciation and model clear articulation (*e.g.*, "Good, c-o-o-k-i-e").

6.   Eventually do not accept poorly articulated responses, but make it as playful as possible (*e.g.*, when the desired object is actually soda, "Oh, you want spinach").

7.   Utilize a receptive discrimination program where Student learns to identify who is articulating clearly and who is not. The person who is articulating poorly should imitate Student's articulation difficulties.

8.   Identify sounds Student is having difficulty with and make them the focus of verbal imitation programs.

Cross-refer: Expressive Labels
Conversation
Communication Temptations

Expressive Labeling

Objectives:

    1.   Provide foundation for building language

    2.   Provide Student with a means to communicate desires

    3.   Provide Student with a means to interact

    4.   Increase Student's understanding and awareness of world around him

Procedure:

The teacher shows an item and asks "What's this?" Initially staff will prompt the response by first having Student point to the object as in Receptive Labeling or by giving a verbal prompt. The prompt will be faded as soon as possible.

IT IS CRITICAL TO SELECT WORDS THAT WOULD BE MOTIVATING TO LEARN (*e.g.*, eat, open, help, no, TV, etc.). IT IS ALSO IMPORTANT TO UTILIZE VARIED INSTRUCTIONS AS QUICKLY AS POSSIBLE (*e.g.*, "Tell me what you see," "what's going on here?," etc.)

Prompts:

Use the Receptive Labeling Program or verbal prompts. Fade the prompt by reducing it to a whisper or only saying the initial sound of the word.

Entry criter:

Student has mastered the items in Matching-Phase 1 or 2 and Receptive Labeling has been attempted. If Receptive Labeling has not been mastered, try doing Expressive Labeling with verbal prompts. It is not necessary to always wait for mastery of Receptive Labeling before starting Expressive.

Mastery crit:

Student performs a response eight out of ten trials correctly with no prompting. This should be repeated with at least one additional teacher.

Phase 1:

Requests. Use objects or pictures that represent items or activities that Student would like to access (*e.g.*, food, drink, play, TV, radio, swinging, etc.). Have Student say what he wants in order to get what he wants. Self-stimulatory objects should be included as a choice. The value of the self-stimulatory object will be diminished by Student choosing other objects (*e.g.*, cookie) over self-stimulatory objects.

Phase 2: **Body parts**.

Developmental Stages
a. Mouth, eyes, nose, feet (B: 2-0)
b. Hair, tongue, head, ears, hands, legs, arms, fingers, stomach, back, teeth, toes (B: 2-6)
c. Chin, thumbs, knees, neck, fingernails (B: 3-6)
d. Heel, ankle, jaw, chest (B: 4-6)
e. Wrist, shoulder, hip, elbow (B: 5-6)
f. Waist (B: 6-6)

Phase 3: **Objects**: toys; animals; clothing; food; household items; furniture. This phase can be started at the same time as Phase 2. Some children find this step easier to learn than body parts.

Phase 4: **Pictures of objects**. The teacher shows a picture of an object and asks, "What's this?"

Phase 5: **Pictures of action**. The teacher shows a picture portraying an action and asks, "What [is/are] [he/they] doing?"

Phase 6: **Actions presented In Vivo**. The teacher demonstrates an action and asks, "What am I doing?"

Phase 7: **Pictures of people**. The teacher shows a picture of a person and asks, "Who is this?"

Phase 8: **People (3-D)**. The teacher points to himself, Student, or another person present and asks, "Who is that?"

Phase 9: **Size** (big/little) (B: 2-6).

Phase 10: **Color**. ("What color?")

Developmental Stages
a. Red, blue (B: 3-6)
b. Green, yellow, orange, purple (B: 4-0)
c. Brown, black, pink, gray (B: 4-6)
d. White (B: 5-6)

Phase 11:   **Shape**. ("What shape?")

Developmental Stages
a.   Circle, square (B: 4-0)
b.   Triangle, rectangle (B: 5-0)
c.   Diamond (B: 6-6)

Phase 12:   **Pictures of places/rooms at home**. The teacher shows pictures of places/rooms and asks Student "What place/room is this?"

Phase 13:   **Places/locations in the community** (actual locations).

Phase 14:   **Emotions**

Phase 15:   **Quantitative Concepts**

Developmental Stages
a.   Many/one (B: 2-6)
b.   Empty/full; light/heavy (B: 3-6)
c.   Short/tall; thin/fat; less/more; short/long (B: 4-0)
d.   Slow/fast; few/many; thin/thick (B: 4-6)
e.   Narrow/wide (B: 5-6)

Next Pgms: Attributes, categories, functions, community helpers, prepositions.

Cross-Refer: Verbal Imitation is a prerequisite. Expressive Labeling leads into Expanding Language I and Conversation-Basic.

Conversation — Basic

Objectives: 1.   Expand use of expressive language

2.   Develop a means for social interaction

3.   Increase social appropriateness

4.   Establish the power of language for controlling people and getting desires met

Procedure: The goal is for Student to learn to use conversational phrases in everyday situations. Initially he will learn to give rote answers in contrived situations. Prompts will be gradually faded as he is expected to use this language in naturally occurring situations.

IT IS CRITICAL TO REALIZE THAT ROTE RESPONSES ARE BEING PROVIDED. HOWEVER, PROVIDING THOUSANDS OF RESPONSES WILL NOT MAKE SOMEONE CONVERSATIONAL. INCREASED OBSERVATIONAL SKILLS, SOCIAL INTERACTION AND EMPHASIS ON BECOMING SOCIAL ARE ESSENTIAL!!!

Phase 1:   **Greeting**. Student should reciprocate when someone says, "Hi." Later this should include saying the person's name.

Phase 2:   **Manding** (directing the behavior of another person)
a.   "Come, [name]" when seeking other person's assistance
b.   "Move, please"
c.   "Give me [object]"
d.   "Let go"
e.   "Come get me" when playing chase
f.   "Go away"
g.   "Quiet down" when someone is too noisy

Phase 3:   **Sentence stems**
a.   "I want . . ."
b.   "It's a . . ."
c.   "That's a . . ."
d.   "I see . . ."
e.   "I have . . ."

Phase 4:   **Commenting**. These are examples of phrases Student should use in various situations to show interest or elicit the interest of another person. The goal is for these to occur unprompted.

    a.   "Here, [name]" (when handing object to person)
    b.   "Look at that!" and points at something interesting.
    c.   "Look [name]" or "Look what I'm doing."
    d.   "There it goes" (as toy is poised to move)
    e.   "I did it!"
    f.   "That's fun"
    g.   "Are you OK?" (when child is hurt)
    h.   "I/We am/are [doing something]." Example: "We are building a BIG sand castle!"

Phase 5:   **Responding**
    a.   "Over there" and points (when asked where something is)
    b.   "What?" (when called by name from distance)
    c.   "Okay" (when asked to do something)
    d.   "Oh," "really," "wow," or "cool" (when someone tells you something)
    e.   "I'm ready"
    f.   "Here I am" (when asked "where are you?")
    g.   "This one" (when asked, "which one do you want?")
    h.   "Come in" (when answering the door)

Assertiveness

Objectives:

1. Help Student identify and meet desires

2. Teach Student to think critically and not automatically accept what someone says

3. Increase ability to function independently and not be reliant on adults (or others) for constant guidance

4. Keep from being victimized

5. Increase awareness

6. Increase spontaneous language

7. Stimulate participation

8. Show that it is okay to be wrong and that Student can be the teacher

9. Help make classroom integration successful

Procedure: Present events that are incorrect and teach Student to verbalize error.

Prompts: Use physical guidance, demonstration, verbal, gestural, voice inflection, or facial expression. Gradually fade the prompts until Student performs independently.

Entry criter: Choice Making (Phase 1 of this program) should be one of the first programs to be taught.

Mastery crit: Student performs a response eight out of ten times correctly with no prompting. This should be repeated with at least one additional teacher.

Phase 1: **Making choices**. This can occur in and out of therapy. In therapy, Student can choose where to sit, what room to work in, what toys to play with, etc. Out of therapy, he can make choices regarding clothes selection, books to read, foods to eat, music to listen to, videos, etc.

Phase 2:   **Playing therapist/teacher**.

Phase 3:   **Expressing displeasure**. Annoy him and teach him to express his displeasure (Examples: "Leave me alone," "Stop it," "No," "It's mine," etc.).

Phase 4:   **Keeping rightful place or object**. Stage event where Student needs to respond physically to assert himself. Take something from him abruptly or get in front of him while waiting for turn. Teach him to make an assertive response (*e.g.*, hold on to item, keep place in line, *etc.*).

Phase 5:   **Conviction**. Make an incorrect statement about something Student knows. For example, incorrectly label an object, action, attribute, etc. He should reject the incorrect information and adhere to the correct label.

Phase 6:   **Make mistakes and have him identify and/or correct mistake** (*e.g.*, throw a toy in the trash)

Phase 7:   **Tell Student to do something inappropriate or impossible and teach him to object** (Example: put a plate in front of him with a block on it and say, "Eat your spaghetti"). Initially, convey the inappropriateness through your voice and then fade the prompt. Start with obvious situations and fade to less obvious ones.

Phase 8:   **Displaying appropriate competitiveness and understanding the concept of winning**. Trying to run fast in a race; trying not to be found in hide and seek; capturing other player's pieces in a game.

Cross-Refer: Communication Temptation

Yes/No

Objectives:

    1.   Provide means for communicating preferences

    2.   Establish choice making

    3.   Promote assertiveness

    4.   Extend understanding and use of basic concepts

    5.   Provide means for answering simple questions

Procedure: The teacher presents an item and asks a question.

Prompts: Use verbal prompts, demonstration, gestural, voice inflection, and/or facial expression to get Student to indicate yes or no. Gradually fade the prompt until Student can respond correctly with no prompt.

Entry criter: Student can attend to relevant stimuli. Student should have identifiable preferences and a means of communicating "yes" and "no" (Examples: verbal, head nod, sign, or pointing).

Mastery crit: Student performs a response eight out of ten times correctly with no prompting. This should be repeated with at least one additional teacher.

Phase 1:   **Desires.** Identify a small group of items that you are sure Student will want and another group of items that Student would not want. Present item that Student likes and ask, "Do you want this?" Immediately prompt Student answers yes and give item to Student. After several successful trials, introduce "no." Show item Student does not like and ask "do you want this?" and immediately prompt Student to say no. As soon as Student says no, remove item from in front of him. After a few successful trials, go back to the "yes" item. The goal is to be able to randomly switch between yes and no questions.

Phase 2:   **Responds to "yes or no" as a prompt for how to answer a question.** ("Do you want juice-yes or no?")

Phase 3:   **Identity of objects** ("Is this a truck?")

Phase 4:   **Identity of persons** ("Is this Mommy?")

Phase 5:   **Actions** ("Is Daddy standing?")

Phase 6:   **Attributes** ("Is this red?")

Phase 7:   **Concepts** ("Is this the corner?")

Phase 8:   **Answers yes/no or true/false questions about things that are not visible** ("Do birds have wings?")

Phase 9:   **Answers yes/no to questions that are partially correct**
(Example: show a green circle and ask if it is a green square)

Negation

Objectives: 1.   Learn to follow one type of instruction

2.   Increase attention to auditory input

3.   Enhance discrimination skills

Phase 1:   **No**. Show Student an item he does not like. Ask him, "Do you want this?"

Phase 2:   **Don't do this**. Demonstrate action and say, "Don't do this." Reinforce for not imitating action.

Phase 3:   **Don't _____**. Teach Student not to perform action when the word "don't" is used (Example: "don't stand"). Reinforce immediately following the verbal direction, before he has a chance to perform the action. If necessary, use hand-over-hand to prevent the action. Gradually lengthen the delay to a few seconds before giving reinforcement and fade out prompting.

Phase 4:   **Say *vs.* Don't Say**.

SD1:   "Say, 'airplane'"
R1:   Student repeats word.

SD2:   "Don't say 'airplane'"
R2:   Student says nothing.

SD3:   Random rotation of SD1 *vs.* SD2

Once Student understands this, change SD to Echo *vs.* Don't Echo. This will allow you to use the phrase "don't echo" to control his unwanted echoing of language.

Phase 5:   **Not _____**. Put out two items, for example, A and B. Ask Student to "Touch Not A." He should touch the other item. Once he understands the concept, change the wording to more natural language, such as, "Show me the one that is not a dog" or "Which one does not have feathers?"

a)   Not [item]: "Show me not ball"

b)   Not [attribute]: "Find not red"

c)   Not [action]: "Which one is not sleeping"

d)   Not [category]: "Find the one that is not an animal"

Joint Attention

Objectives:

1. Increase Student's awareness of the environment and the activities of others

2. Teach him how to get another person's attention

3. Increase his desire to direct and obtain the attention of others

Prompts: Use physical guidance, demonstration, verbal, pointing or position prompt. Gradually fade the prompts until Student performs independently.

Entry criter: Phase 1 can be started as soon as Student has mastered Nonverbal Imitation.

Mastery crit: Student performs a response nine out of ten times correctly with no prompting with two choices; eight out of ten times with three or more choices. This should be repeated with at least one additional teacher.

Procedure: Teach Student to be aware of whether another person is attending and how to get another person to attend.

Phase 1: **Ask Student, "Where is [object]?"** He answers "over there" and points in the direction of the item.

Phase 2: **Tell Student to give an object to a certain person.** That person should not attend to him and not accept object until he says, "Here, [name]." Do this also with throwing a ball. He should say "Catch, [name]" before person attempts to catch his throw.

Phase 3: **Getting a person's attention.** Tell Student to tell or ask a person something. That person should be unresponsive to his initial attempts to communicate. He should be prompted to repeat the person's name and tug at the person's arm.

Phase 4: **Showing off something that he made.** Make sure other person can see it.

Phase 5:   **Identifying where a person is pointing.**

      a.   The teacher points at something and says, "Student, go over there."

      b.   The teacher asks Assistant "Where is the cookie?" Assistant points and says, "over there." The teacher tells Student to go get the cookie.

      c.   The assistant points at something. The teacher asks Student, "What is Assistant pointing to?"

Phase 6:   **Identifying where a person is looking.** The assistant looks at something. Ask Student, "what is Assistant looking at?"

Phase 7:   **Identifying the direction of movement.** Put toy animals in a line and face them in a certain direction. Ask Student where they are going. He should point in the proper direction.

Phase 8:   **Identifying whether a person can hear him.** Have Student say something to Assistant, who is either close by or in another part of the house. Ask Student whether Assistant can hear. He can judge this based not only on the distance, but also whether the assistant has responded.

Phase 9:   **Identifying whether a person can see him.** Ask student about something that is visible to him. Have an Assistant either close by or in another part of the house. Ask Student whether Assistant can see item. He can judge this based on whether Assistant is nearby and is looking in the right direction.

Phase10:   **Identifying whether a person knows some information.** Stage an event while Assistant is either close by or in another part of the house. Ask Student whether Assistant could know what happened. He can judge this based on either Assistant having seen an event or having heard something that was said.

Phase 11:   **Do unusual things to get Student to comment.** Some of these procedures were described by Margery Rappoport in Maurice et al. (1996).

      a.   Wear a wig

      b.   Wear glasses upside down

      c.   "Accidentally" color on the table. Model saying, "uh-oh"

      d.   Drop materials off the table. Model says, "fall down"

e.   Attempt to put his shoe on his hand

f.   Put a hammer in the silverware drawer

g.   Put a bunch of celery in the clothes hamper

h.   Rearrange the furniture or remove something obvious from the environment

i.   Each take several turns at a turn-taking routine, then do something unexpected

Cross-Refer: Basic Conversation
Communication Temptations
Expanding Language I
Describing
Assertiveness

Emotions

Objectives:

1. Identify emotional states

2. Develop empathy

3. Facilitate social interactions

4. Identify potential ways to change emotional states

5. Develop understanding of cause and effect

Procedure:

Present different emotions to Student, either through role-playing or through pictures, to teach the identification of feelings, possible causes and how to alter the situation.

Assemble a variety of picture cards that clearly portray basic emotions. (Lakeshore publishes a Feelings and Faces Game.)

Beginning Emotions	**Advanced Emotions**
Happy	Frustrated
Sad	Nervous
Angry	Excited
	Confused
Intermediate	Bored
Scared	Worried
Surprised	Jealous
Tired	Proud
Silly	Embarrassed
*Hungry/thirsty	
Sick	

*Note that these feelings are determined situationally or behaviorally, rather than by facial expression.

MAKE SURE EMOTIONS ARE AGE-APPROPRIATE (*E.G.*, A FOUR-YEAR OLD WOULD NOT UNDERSTAND BORED)

Phase 1:   **Non-identical matching of emotions in pictures**. Put pictures of a model showing two or more different emotions on the table. Show Student a picture of a different model showing the same emotion and tell him to "put with same."

Phase 2:   **Receptive labeling of emotions in pictures**. Choose one emotion to start the training and use the others as distractors. Put out a picture of emotion one and a picture of the distractor emotion. Tell Student, "Touch [emotion]" and prompt as needed. Once he has mastered emotion one, teach emotion two. Then conduct random trials of the two emotions. Add additional emotions as each is mastered.

Phase 3:   **Expressive labeling of emotions in pictures**. Show Student a picture and ask, "How does he feel?"

Phase 4:   **Demonstrating emotions**. Use imitation to teach Student to demonstrate various emotions.

Phase 5:   **Recognizing emotions of others portrayed in vivo**. Demonstrate a facial expression and ask Student, "How do I feel?"

Phase 6:   **Labeling his own emotions**. Contrive a situation where Student would be experiencing a certain emotion. This can be done through role-play or nonverbal imitation. Ask him, "How do you feel?"

Phase 7:   **Identifying causes for emotions**. Use pictures that portray cause and effect or stage vignettes. Ask Student why he feels a certain way or why another person feels a certain way.

Generalize to the natural environment, looking for naturally occurring opportunities to review emotions.

Teacher: How does your sister feel?
Student: She's sad.
Teacher: Why is she sad?
Student: Because she can't have the toy.

Teacher: How do you feel right now?
Student: Happy!
Teacher: Why?
Student: Because you're tickling me!

Phase 8:   **Making someone feel a certain emotion**. Set up a situation where a person is feeling a certain way. Instruct Student to "make [person] feel [emotion]" (*e.g.*, make someone feel happy by giving them a hug).

Phase 9:   **Generalize to naturally occurring situations**. Have Student describe how he is feeling or how another person is feeling.

Phase 10:   **Empathy**. Demonstrates knowledge of how to respond to situation.

Examples: someone says and/or acts:

Cold	Frightened
Hungry	Sad
Injured	Angry

Student either explains what he would do or demonstrates an appropriate response.

Cross-Refer: Matching
Receptive Labels
Expressive Labels

Gestures (Pragmatics)

Objectives:

1. Develop an understanding of often-used nonverbal communications

2. Increase environmental awareness

3. Increase ability to read social cues

4. Improve classroom and group functioning

5. Develop additional means of communicating

Prompts: Use physical guidance, demonstration, verbal, pointing or position prompt. Gradually fade the prompts until Student performs independently.

Mastery crit: Student performs a response nine out of ten times correctly. This should be repeated with at least one additional teacher.

Phase 1: **Student imitates gestures**

Gesture	Meaning
Extend arm; move palm up	Stand up
Beckon with finger or hand	Come here
Arm outstretched, palm outward	Stop
Index finger raised	Wait a minute
Wave arm back and forth	Move
Wag finger	Don't do that
Shrug shoulders	I don't know
Finger over lips	Be quiet
Applause/thumbs up	Good job
Two thumbs up	Great job!
OK sign	OK
Pat tummy	Delicious
Yuck; tongue out	Bad taste
Pinch nose	Bad smell
Chin in hand	Bored
Shift feet; look at watch	I want to go

Lean forward; nod	Interested
Roll eyes	That's ridiculous
Yawn	Tired
Cross arms	Frustrated
Rub chin/forehead between thumb and fingers	Thinking
Tap forehead with the front of the wrist	I forgot/I messed up

Phase 2:   **Student performs gesture on request.** Teacher says, "Use gestures, to tell me . . ."

Phase 3:   **Teacher demonstrates a gesture and asks, "What does this mean?"**

Phase 4:   **Student demonstrates the response in the appropriate context.**

    a.   Indicating where someone or something is located by pointing. May be accompanied with narrative phrases including "It's over there" or "on the shelf"

    b.   Indicating something tastes good by rubbing his tummy

    c.   Indicating he knows an answer or desires an item or turn. For example, in response to the question "Who wants ice cream?," he raises his hand stating "I do" or without verbal response

    d.   Shaking his head "no" and nodding "yes" when appropriate

    e.   Acting bored by putting his chin in his hand

    f.   Expressing emotion. Example: he crosses his arms to communicate frustration

    g.   Pulling the torso back and making a face when creepy, yucky items are presented. Example: "Yuck, bug soup"

Phase 5:   **Student reads the nonverbal cue and adjusts behavior accordingly.**

    a.   Student walks forward or takes a turn when the teacher beckons with finger or points

    b.   Student steps back or moves backward in response to underhanded wave

c. Reading a head nod or a shake accurately. The teacher may set up a situation where a model tastes a food and he is asked if he liked it

d. Reading pointing gestures to indicate where desired items are located, or where Student should sit or stand during an activity

c. Using two models (or pictures) indicating which person is listening (leaning forward, looking at the person, perhaps nodding) and which is not paying attention (looking away, looking at her fingernails, reading a book)

Cross-Refer: Joint Attention
Emotions
Pretend Actions

Attributes

Objectives:
1. Expand language

2. Increase understanding of concepts

3. Increase awareness of environment

Procedure: Follow basic discrimination training procedure. Use concrete items to represent each attribute. Select items that are as similar as possible and vary only on the attribute being taught. Each concept can be taught first as matching, then as receptive discrimination, and as expressive label. Student may learn better first using objects and then pictures. However, he may be able to learn readily going directly to pictures. In either case, the concept needs to be generalized using a wide range of materials.

Prompts: Use verbal, gestural or position prompt. Gradually fade the prompts until Student performs independently.

Entry criter: Start with concrete attributes and move to the abstract. Refer to developmental norms for age-appropriate language.

Mastery crit: Student performs a response nine out of ten times correctly with no prompting with two choices, eight out of ten times with three or more choices. This should be repeated with at least one additional teacher.

Phase 1: **Color**

Phase 2: **Size**

Phase 3: **Physical attributes.** "Touch [hot]" *vs.* "touch [cold]".
a. Hot/cold
b. Wet/dry
c. Rough/smooth
d. Hard/soft
e. Sharp/dull
f. Light/heavy
g. Sweet/sour
h. Dark/light

       i.   Clean/dirty
       j.   Old/new
       k.   Straight/crooked

Phase 4:   **Gender.** Use pictures of boys and girls.
       a.   Matching: "put boy with boys" *vs.* "put girl with girls"
       b.   Receptive: "touch boy" *vs.* "touch girl"

Phase 5:   **Composition.** Receptive: "touch [plastic]." Expressive: "What is this made of?"
       a.   Plastic
       b.   Wood
       c.   Paper
       d.   Cloth
       e.   Metal
       f.   Leather
       g.   Glass

Phase 6:   **Temporal**
       a.   First/last
       b.   Before/after

Phase 7:   **Spatial.** "Show me [near]" *vs.* "show me [far]"
       a.   Up/down
       b.   Around
       c.   Near/far
       d.   Middle

Phase 8:   **Quantitative.** "Roll the ball fast" *vs.* "roll the ball slow."
       a.   Fast/slow
       b.   Long/short
       c.   Tall/short
       d.   Thin/wide
       e.   Part/half/whole
       f.   All/some/none
       g.   Few/many
       h.   Light/heavy
       i.   Empty/full

Phase 9:   **Other Opposites**
       a.   Night/day
       b.   Open/closed
       c.   Young/old
       d.   On/off (light, shoes)

Phase 10:   **Logical connectors**
            a.   Or: "Give me a blue one or a red one"
            b.   And: "Give me a blue one and a red one"
            c.   Not: "Give me one that is not blue"

Functions

Objectives:	1. Increase understanding of the everyday world
	2. Expand language
	3. Improve memory and reasoning skills
Procedure:	Items are presented to Student and he is asked to explain the function or vice versa.
Prompts:	Use physical guidance, demonstration, verbal, pointing or position prompt. Gradually fade the prompts until Student performs independently.
Entry criter:	Expressive Labels. Expressive Actions.
Mastery crit:	Student performs a response nine out of ten times correctly with no prompting. This should be repeated with at least one additional teacher.

Phase 1:   **Nonverbal (live action)**

      a.   Show an object to Student. Ask, "What do you do with this?" Student should demonstrate an appropriate action.

      b.   Put several objects on the table. Teacher pantomimes an action and asks, "What do you use for this?" Student should choose the appropriate object.

Phase 2:   **Place a number of 3-D objects on the table**

      a.   (Picture SD) Show Student an action picture and ask, "What would you need for this?" He chooses an object from the table. (This could also be done as a matching task by asking, "Where does this go?" and allowing him to place the action picture with the corresponding object).

      b.   (Verbal SD) Ask Student what you would use to: brush your teeth, wash your face, drink your juice, etc. He chooses an object from the table.

Phase 3:   **Show Student a 3-D object and ask "what is this for?"**

     a.   (Nonverbal response) Student chooses the correct action picture from the choices on the table.

     b.   (Verbal response) Student tells what the object is used for.

Phase 4:   **Place several 2-D pictures of items on the table**

     a.   (Picture SD) Show Student an action picture and ask, "What would you need for this?" He chooses object from table. (This could also be done as a matching task by asking, "Where does this go?" and allowing him to place the action picture with the corresponding object.)

     b.   (Verbal SD) Ask Student what you would use to: brush your teeth, wash your face, drink your juice, etc. He chooses correct picture from table.

Phase 5:   **Show Student a 2-D picture and ask "what is this for?"**

     a.   Nonverbal action response: Student simulates the action that would be performed.

     b.   Nonverbal multiple choice: Student chooses the correct action picture from choices on the table.

     c.   Verbal response: Student tells what the item is used for.

Phase 6:   **Intra-verbal 1 (No visual cues are used).** Ask Student what you would use to: brush your teeth, wash your face, drink your juice, etc. Student gives a verbal response.

Phase 7:   **Intra-verbal 2 (No visual cues are used).** Ask Student what a [toothbrush, soap, cup, etc.] is used for. Student gives a verbal response.

     a.   Chairs, cars, beds (B: 2-0)
     b.   Houses, pencils, dishes (B: 2-6)
     c.   Books, telephones, scissors (B: 3-0)

Phase 8:   **Function of body parts**

     a.   "What do you do with your eyes?"
     b.   "What do you see with?"

Phase 9: **Function of rooms**

a. "What do you do in [room]?"
b. "Where do you [action]?"

Cross-Refer: General Knowledge and Reasoning
Categories

Categories

Objectives: 1.   Make associations of things that are related

2.   Expand communication

3.   Develop abstract reasoning

Procedure: Select groups of items that are related. Start with simple categories like animals, food, and clothing. It will usually work to use pictures of items. Some children may need to have this first presented with 3-D items.

Examples:
Animals, food, clothes, furniture, transportation/vehicles, toys, rooms, tools, shapes, letters, numbers, fruit, drink, objects in the sky, plants, objects in the ocean, body parts, people, instruments, things in the cupboard, things in the kitchen, things in the garage, etc.

Prompts: Use physical guidance, demonstration, verbal prompts, pointing, or a combination. Gradually fade prompts so that Student is performing independently.

Entry criter.   Student has completed non-identical matching and object-to-picture matching.

Mastery crit: Student performs a response eight out of ten times correctly with no prompting. This should be repeated with at least one additional teacher.

Phase 1:   **Matching**. Student sorts items into piles. Put out one picture for each category to be sorted and label the category of the picture. Then give him additional pictures one at a time and tell him to "put with [animal]." Once he is performing consistently, this can be turned into a sorting task by giving him a pile of mixed up pictures and telling him to sort them.

Phase 2:   **Receptive**. Put out two or more pictures, each representing a different category. Tell him to "give me [animal]."

Phase 3:   **Expressive**. Show him a picture and ask, "What is this?" Student should answer by naming the item (*e.g.*, cow). Then ask, "What is cow?" and he should name the category animal.

Phase 4:   **Naming**. Ask him to name something from the category (*e.g.*, "Name an animal"). After he names one item, praise him and ask him to name another item (*e.g.*, "Name ANOTHER animal"). If prompting is necessary, put pictures of various categories out on table, including the category being requested.

Phase 5:   **Complex categories**. Ask him to name something that meets two or more requirements. Examples: "Name an animal that lives in the ocean"; "Name a food you would eat for breakfast"; "Name a vehicle that does not go on the road."

General Knowledge And Reasoning I

Objectives:

1. Teach Student general information that is **functional and age appropriate**

2. Develop abstract reasoning

3. Increase awareness of environment

4. Provide means for expanding language

5. Increase ability to answer questions

Procedure: Ask Student questions regarding general information. Provide him the information if he does not know the answer.

IT IS CRITICAL TO REALIZE THAT COMPREHENSION IS UNLIKELY TO BE DEVELOPED BY PROVIDING NUMEROUS BITS OF UNRELATED INFORMATION. COMPREHENSION IS DEVELOPED THROUGH TEACHING RELATED EXAMPLES OF A CONCEPT UNTIL STUDENT IS ABLE TO GENERATE NEW EXAMPLES ON HIS OWN.

A. Associations

1. 3-D object matching (items that go together). Present one item and ask, "What goes with this?" Student selects an item or picture from several choices on the table.

2. 2-D picture matching.

Associations

Pencil/paper	Shovel/pail
Sock/shoe	Spoon/bowl
Pillow/bed	Toothbrush/toothpaste
Napkin/plate	Coat/hat
Swimsuit/towel	Lunchbox/sandwich
Chalk/chalkboard	Scissors/paper
Flowers/vase	Tape/tape player
Videocassette/VCR	Shirt/pants
Glove/hand	Sock/foot

Ball/bat	Candles/birthday cake
Paints/brush	Bike/helmet
Basketball/hoop	Broom/dustpan
Pitcher/cup	Hairbrush/hair dryer
Soap/washcloth	Train/track
Baby/bottle	Crayon/coloring book
Nut/bolt	Hammer/nail
Lawnmower/grass	Vacuum/rug

B.   Auditory Discrimination - Live Sound. Put items on the table that make a sound. Examples: squeeze toy, maraca, bell, toy police car with siren. Present a sound and say "find same." To prompt, make sound with item in view of Student. He will imitate the action and make the same sound. Fade prompt by making sound with item out of view.

    1.   Chooses from objects

    2.   Chooses from pictures

    3.   Gives an answer with no visual choices

C.   Auditory Discrimination - recorded sound

    1.   Chooses from objects

    2.   Chooses from pictures

    3.   Gives an answer with no visual choices.

D.   Associates action with person, character or animal

    1.   What does a person, character or animal say? (Cow says 'moo')

    2.   What does a person, character or animal eat? (Winnie the Pooh eats honey)

    3.   What does a person, character or animal do? (Pirates hunt for buried treasure)

    4.   Who/what says [sound]?

    5.   Who eats [item]?

    6.   Who [does action]?

E. Identifies locations

   1. Rooms in his house
      a. Receptive photo I.D.
      b. Expressive photo labels
      c. Goes to named room/location
      d. Names room/location where he is

   2. Generic rooms (from magazines, books, etc.)

   3. Locations in community (park, post office, McDonald's, etc.)

F. Occupations/Community Helpers/Characters

   1. Receptive identification of a person
   2. "Who [does role]?" - points to picture
   3. Expressive labeling of person
   4. "Who [does role]?" - verbal response
   5. "What does a [person] do?"
   6. "Where would you see [person]?" - points to picture
   7. "Where would you see [person]?" - verbal response
   8. "What does a [person] use?" - points to picture
   9. "What does a [person] use?" - verbal response

G. Opposites

   1. Putting items together.

   2. Receptive: Teacher puts out two or more pictures on table and asks, "What is the opposite of . . .?" Student points to the correct picture.

   3. Expressive: Teacher asks, "What is the opposite of . . .?" Student answers. No visual is provided.

H. Composition: "What is it made of?" (wood, paper, glass, metal, etc.)

   1. Matching. Puts together items made of the same material.

   2. Receptively identifies the item that is made of the material.

      SD: "Point to wood"
      R: Points to an item made of wood

3.   Names material that item is made of
        SD: Show shirt. Ask student, "What is this made of?"
        R: "Cloth"

General Knowledge And Reasoning II

Objectives:

1. Teach Student general information that is **functional and age appropriate**

2. Develop more abstract reasoning

Procedure: Ask Student questions regarding general information. Provide him with the information if he does not know the answer.

IT IS CRITICAL TO REALIZE THAT COMPREHENSION IS UNLIKELY TO BE DEVELOPED BY PROVIDING NUMEROUS BITS OF UNRELATED INFORMATION. COMPREHENSION IS DEVELOPED THROUGH TEACHING RELATED EXAMPLES OF A CONCEPT UNTIL STUDENT IS ABLE TO GENERATE NEW EXAMPLES ON HIS OWN.

A. Identification/Describing. For this program, you should generate five or more examples as responses to each item. Ask Student to give you a certain number of responses starting with two, and gradually expanding it, but do not ask for more than is developmentally reasonable. When you are prompting him, you should randomize the order and which ones you give him so that his responses do not become rote. Be sure to very heavily reinforce any variations that he generates on his own.

1. Describes person or object (person/item not present).

2. Identifies person or object with certain characteristics (person/item not present).

3. What do you _____ (cook on, drive in, etc.)?

4. Where would you find a _____ (bed, stove, steering wheel, cloud, etc.)?

5. What would you see in a _____ (kitchen, library, doctor's office, etc.)?

B.   Associations II

    1.   Verbal question - verbal response.

        SD: "What goes with shoe?"
        R: "Sock"

    2.   Why do these go together?

        SD: "How does a shoe and a sock go together?"
        R: "I wear socks on my feet"

C.   Reasoning: Can explain why we take certain action

    1.   Why do we take a bath? Why do you go to the doctor?

D.   Knows what to do in different situations ("What do you when you are?")

    1.   Sleepy, cold, tired, hungry, cut your finger, sick (B: 3-0)

    2.   See your shoe is untied, are thirsty, want to go outside and it is raining (B: 4-0)

E.   Knows where to go for various things

    1.   Where do we go to mail a letter?

F.   Impossible Tasks

    1.   Can you touch the ceiling? Why not?

G.   Irregularities/Absurdities. Present actual items that have something wrong or use pictures.

    1.   Identification: Student points out the thing that is wrong.
    2.   Explaining: Student says what the problem is. Example: the car has three wheels
    3.   Correcting: Student fixes it or describes what should be done. Example: he assembles Mr. Potato Head the proper way

H.   Identifying item missing in a picture

I.   Riddles

J. Analogies (An elephant is big; a mouse is _____)

K. Extending Patterns: ABCABCA . . . . What comes next?

L. Coding. Student is presented with a legend (*e.g.*, Heart=A, Star=B, Circle=C, etc.). He is then given a grid that has one part of the code and room to put the translation.

Same vs. Different

Objectives:
1. Increase abstract reasoning

2. Increase awareness and attention to detail of objects in the environment

Procedure: Present items that are alike on a certain dimension and one additional item that is different on that dimension. Start with obvious physical characteristics and progress to more abstract attributes and finely detailed differences.

Prompts: Use demonstration, verbal, pointing or position prompt. Gradually fade the prompts until Student performs independently.

Entry criter: Matching is a prerequisite.

Mastery crit: Student performs a response eight out of ten times correctly with no prompting over two consecutive sessions. This should be repeated with at least one additional teacher.

Phase 1: **Have a group of objects that are identical (*e.g.*, all same color) and place one object in the group that differs on that dimension.** Ask Student to give you the object that is different. Once he understands, gradually reduce the field until there are two items that are the same and one that is different. Then, on each trial after he has given you the different one (there will be two identical items left on table), tell him to give you "same." It may be necessary to prompt him to pick up both of the items and hand them to you. Gradually start randomizing the order in which you ask for the same or different items.

Phase 2: **Find same/find different**. Put two items on the table (*e.g.*, an apple and a shoe). Show him a shoe and ask him to find the one that is the same/ different.

Phase 3: **Expressive**. Put out two items. Ask Student, "Are these the same or different?"

Generalize into the natural environment (*e.g.*, during games, chores, Playdoh, etc.). Examples: "Bring me the same plate." "Pick a different one." "Color yours the same as mine." "Make yours different."

Phase 4: **Follow the above procedure and ask Student "Why are they different?" or "Why are they the same?"** He answers, "Because they're both shoes" (same) or "because this one's a shoe and this one is an apple" (different).

Phase 5: **Use items that are the same in one respect, but different in another way**. Student needs to answer both "how are they the same?" and "how are they different?" Examples: a red block and a green block; two animals; a crayon and a pencil; etc.

Attribute
Category
Function

Cross-Refer: Matching

Prepositions

Objectives:

1. Teach Student the relationship between objects and the environment

2. Teach him a building block of language

3. Provide him with a means to find or place objects in the environment

4. Teach the concept of "where"

Procedure:

This is a program that children often find difficult and can become quite aversive. If you do not have early success, you may want to defer it for a while.

It is important to make this a fun drill. Be creative in the use of objects and the method of presentation. For example, make this into a zoo game and use a cage to put animals in, on, beside, etc. Other examples:

> Farmyard game with animals and tractor
> Castle with figures
> Ocean scene
> Doll house
> School bus

Select an item such as a box, a cup, or a bucket (referred to as the stationary item). The item must have at least two different prepositions that can be used with it. For example, in the right side up position, a cup can be used for in and beside. In the upside down position, it can be used for on, under, and beside. Use a movable item such as a block or small toy to put in the various locations such as on, under, etc. The item should be varied frequently as you are doing the trials. This can also be done by having Student place the movable item in reference to a chair or table (*e.g.,* put Elmo under the table).

Once this is mastered at the table, generalize the concepts to picture books, locations around the house, and outside.

Phase 1:   **Matching pictures**. Use pictures that depict various positional concepts (*e.g.*, a child on top *vs.* under a table). Put two pictures out showing the same person in different locations. Give Student a picture of a different person in one of the locations and say "put with [on top]."

Phase 2:   **a)** [OPTIONAL] **As a first step, it may be helpful to teach the concept of top *vs.* the side of an object**. Put the stationary item in front of Student and ask him to touch to top *vs.* side. Use the basic discrimination training paradigm. Prompt using a dramatic slapping gesture to model and encourage him to have fun with the activity.

b) Teach Student to place a movable object on top *vs.* beside the stationary object. Use interesting figures as the movable objects and use a different object every few trials. Additional receptive prepositions should be introduced once on top and beside are mastered:

Receptive Prepositions - Beginning Level
On top   Beside
In   Under

Receptive Prepositions - Advanced Level
Behind   In front
Next to   Between

A way to make this interesting to him is to use a favorite character. Have the character ask him for directions to a location in reference to some stationary object (*e.g.*, "Excuse me, can you show me how to get behind the chair?"). Student can make or watch the character "walk" to the location.

Another idea is to use Colorforms. Tell Student to put a form in a certain location (*e.g.*, put Batman in the Batmobile; put Mickey under the table).

Preposition game: Use a chair or some other object that has clear positions (*e.g.*, on, under, behind, etc.). Then place inverted cups in these various locations and hide a treat under one of them. Tell Student to look on/under/behind the chair. If he goes to the correct cup he gets the treat that is hidden there.

For in front and behind, be sure to use items that have an absolute front and back. A chair is okay; a box is not. This can also be done with two animals lined up head to tail. Ask Student to point to who's in front *vs.* behind.

For generalization, you can have him go on a treasure hunt with treats hidden in various locations: on, under, in, etc.

Phase 3:   **Have Student place himself in various locations in reference to stationary items.** Examples: "Go under the table," "Stand on the chair," "Go in the laundry basket," "Go behind mommy."

Phase 4:   **Receptive discrimination of prepositions in pictures**

Phase 5:   **Expressive 3-D**. Using a stationary and a movable objects, demonstrate the various prepositions and ask Student "where is the [movable object]?"

Phase 6:   **Expressive 2-D**. Use pictures to present concepts. Curious George books work well for this step.

Pronouns

Objectives:
1. Teach the relationship between himself and the environment

2. Teach him a building block of language

3. Promote language that sounds more appropriate (i.e., eliminating pronoun reversal)

4. Teach concept of "who"

Procedure:
Initially, Student will be taught to receptively respond to pronouns. The teacher will direct Student to touch his own or the teacher's body part (e.g., "Touch your nose.") Prompting may consist of the teacher using Student's name as part of the instruction and slowly fading it out until only the pronoun is provided. For example, "Touch my-**TEACHER'S** nose" or "Touch your-**STUDENT'S** hand." At the beginning of training, you should vary the body part very infrequently. As he gets better at the pronouns, you can vary the body part more frequently. Once this is mastered, move on to expressive use of pronouns.

It may be helpful to use inanimate objects, such as a stuffed animal or characters (e.g., Mickey Mouse's nose vs. teacher's nose). Peers or dolls may be used to teach third person pronouns such as his and hers.

Expressive and receptive programs for first and second person pronouns (e.g., I, you) are not to be mixed until each element is independently mastered. This is to reduce confusion over pronoun reversal.

Entry criter:
Student has mastered body parts and Expanding Language I, using at least two word phrases. (The description of Expanding Language I is in the next section). For a nonverbal student, he should have mastered receptive discrimination of object/attribute combinations.

Mastery crit:
Student performs a response nine out of ten times correctly. This should be repeated with at least one additional teacher.

Phase 1:   **Receptive Pronouns - Possessive ("Point to _____ nose")**

    a. John's (Teacher's) vs. Student's
    b. My-**JOHN**'s (Teacher's) vs. Your-**Student**'s
    c. **MY**-John's (Teacher's) vs. **YOUR**-Student's
    d. My vs. Your
    e. His vs. Her - persons
    f. His vs. Her - pictures
    g. Their/Our/Your (plural) - persons
    h. Their/Our/Your (plural) - pictures
    i. This/That/These/Those

For this step, you can use items besides body parts. For example put candies on the table. One is "my candy" and one is "your candy." The teacher may say "Eat **MY** candy." If Student is correct, he gets to eat the candy.

Phase 2:   **Receptive Pronouns - Objects**

    a. Me vs. You ("Point to me")
    b. Him vs. Her ("Give [object] to her")

Phase 3:   **Expressive Pronouns.** The teacher will touch either Student's or staff's own body part or clothing, and ask "Whose [body part]?"

    a. Possessive - My vs. Your
        Teacher: Whose nose?
        Student: My nose.

    b. Possessive - His vs. Her
        Teacher: Whose shoe?
        Student: Her shoe.

    c. Possessive - Their vs. Our (with teams)
        Teacher: Whose ball?
        Student: Their ball.

    d. Nominative - He vs. She
        Teacher: What's happening?
        Student: He is _____

    e. Nominative - I vs. You
        Teacher: Who has the ball?
        Student: I do

f.   Nominative - They vs. We

g.   Nominative/Possessive combinations ("You are touching my nose.")

h.   This/That/These/Those

Expanding Language

Objectives:

1. Facilitate language that is not teacher directed—beginning of spontaneous speech

2. Facilitate conversational skills

3. Increase the fluency, fluidity and length of verbal production

4. Increase awareness and attending

Procedure:

Initially, the items will be 3-D and will be presented as discrete items. Use items from Expressive Labeling. The teacher presents an item and elicits from Student a description of what he sees. Initially, the teacher may ask a question such as, "What do you see?" But it is preferable to teach him to comment without needing to be asked a question. In the beginning, just have him name the item. Then the program is expanded by presenting two or more items and also moving into 2-D representation. The desired response is a description of what the person is doing or what is happening in the picture. Next, books or complex pictures with multiple concepts will be utilized. Finally, objects will be pointed out in the environment. To systematically increase Student's ability to comment on complex scenes, you can take pictures starting with single discrete items and gradually increase the number of items included in the scene. Videotape can be used as an additional medium to present stimulus material.

The eventual goal is for Student to provide a detailed description (*i.e.*, multiple descriptors), with as little prompting from teacher as possible. Fade from verbal prompts to nonverbal communications (*e.g.*, leaning in and motioning with the hand to prompt more verbiage). This speeds generalizations in the natural environment and increases interpersonal attending skills.

Entry criter:

Student has mastered items in Phase 3 of Expressive Labeling.

Mastery crit:

Student performs a response eight out of ten times correctly with no prompting. This should be repeated with at least one additional teacher.

Phase 1:   **"What's this?"**

      a.   One-word answer. Show item to Student and ask a question.

              SD: "What's this?"
              R: "[object name]"

      b.   Student answers in a sentence

              SD: "What's this?"
              R: "It's a [object name]"

Phase 2:   **"What do you see?"**

      a.   Single 3-D object on table

              SD: "What do you see?"
               R: "I see [object]"

      b.   Multiple 3-D objects on the table

              SD: "What do you see?"
               R: "I see [object] and [object] . . ."

      c.   Single 3-D object around the room, looking out the window, or standing outside

              SD: "What do you see?" (may be accompanied by pointing gesture, which is later faded if appropriate)
              R: "I see [object]"

      d.   Multiple 3-D objects around the room, looking out the window, or standing outside

              SD: "What do you see?"
               R: "I see [object] and [object] . . ."

      e.   Single 2-D picture on the felt board ("I see [object]")

      f.   Multiple 2-D pictures on the felt board ("I see [object] and [object] . . .")

      g.   Names single item in a complex picture such as a scene from a story book ("I see [object]")

      h.   Names multiple items in a complex picture such as a scene from a story book ("I see [object] and [object]")

Phase 3:   **Verbs - (one-word answer).** You may have Student respond without the "-ing" ending if it makes it easier for him, but all staff should be consistent in the response they accept.

> SD: "What is [person] doing?"
> R: "Sleeping"; "Eating"; "Running"; etc.

Phase 4:   **Verb/object combinations - "What is [person] doing?"**
Examples: riding bike, kicking ball

Phase 5:   **Subject/verb combinations**
a.   Noun as subject

> SD: "What is Mommy doing?"
> R: "Mommy is standing"

b.   Pronoun as subject

> SD: "What is he doing?"
> R: "He is sleeping"

c.   Student supplies pronoun

> SD: "What's happening (in the picture)?"
> R: "IIe is sleeping"

Phase 6:   **Adjective/Object - answers in a phrase**

> SD: "What is it?"
> R: "Yellow truck"

Phase 7:   **Adjective/Adjective/Object - answers in a phrase**

> SD: "What is it?"
> R: "Big red ball"

Phase 8:   **Subject/verb/object combinations**
a.   Noun as subject

> SD: "What is (the) girl doing?"
> R: "(The) girl is kissing (the) baby"

  b. Student supplies noun

    SD: "What's happening (in the picture)?"
    R: "(The) girl is kissing (the) baby"

  c. Pronoun as subject

    SD: "What is she doing?"
    R: "She is kicking (a) ball"

  d. Student supplies pronoun

    SD: "What's happening (in the picture)?"
    R: "She is kicking (a) ball"

Phase 9:   **Adjective/Object - answers in a sentence**
  a. "What is it?" ("It's a yellow truck")
  b. "What do you see?" ("I see a big ball")
  c. "What do you have?" ("I have a brown horse")

Phase 10:   **Adjective/Adjective/Object - answers in a sentence**
  a. "What is it?" ("It's a little yellow truck")
  b. "What do you see?" ("I see big red ball")
  c. "What do you have?" ("I have a big brown horse")

Phase 11:   **Adjective/Object/Preposition/Object**
  Example: blue truck on table

Phase 12:   **Subject/verb/object/descriptor combinations**

Phase 13:   **Generalize language to everyday situations**

Cross-Refer: Communication Temptations
       Conversation-Basic
       Expressive Labels
       "I Spy" game

Verb Tenses

Objectives:
1. Provide Student with language for describing events in the past, and for anticipating events that will occur in the future

2. Increase his awareness of the temporal relationship of events

Procedure: Ask Student questions about actions in various tenses. Use live action or pictures.

Prompts: Use physical guidance, demonstration, verbal, pointing or position prompt. Gradually fade the prompts until Student performs independently.

Entry criter: Student has mastered expressive verbs.

Mastery crit: Student performs a response nine out of ten times with no prompting. This should be repeated with at least one additional teacher.

Phase 1: **Present tense**.

SD1: "[person] is _____ing."

SD2: Show a picture of an action. "What's happening?"
R2: "[person] is _____ing."

SD3: Demonstrate an action. "What am I doing?"
R3: "You are _____ing."

SD4a: Demonstrate an action. "Do this."
R4a: Imitates the action.
SD4b: Teacher ceases the action as soon as Student starts; have him continue to perform the action. "What are you doing?"
R4b: "I am _____ing."

Phase 2: **Past tense**. Start with regular verbs, then teach irregular verbs.

SD1a: Demonstrate an action. "Do this."
R1a: Imitates the action.

SD1b: Teacher ceases the action as soon as Student starts; have him continue to perform the action. "What are you doing?"

R1b: "I am _____ing."

SD1c: Have Student cease the action. Pause. "What **DID** you do?"
(Emphasis on **DID** is a prompt to be faded out as Student learns concept.)

R1c: "I _____ed."

SD2:   Random rotation of past *vs.* present tense questions with Student performing actions.

R2:   Student answers using correct verb tense.

SD3a: Use a stuffed animal, doll or other character. Have character perform an action. "What is [character] doing?"

R3a: "[character] is _____ing."

SD3b: Have character stop action. Pause. "What did [character] do?"

R3b: "[character] _____ed."

SD4:   Random rotation of past *vs.* present tense questions with characters performing actions.

R4:   Student answers using correct verb tense.

SD5a: Show a picture of an action. "What is [person] doing?"

R5a: "[person] is _____ing."

SD5b: Tip picture down. Pause. "What did [person] do?"

R5b: "[person] _____ed."

SD6:   Random rotation of past *vs.* present tense questions with characters performing actions.

R6:   Student answers using correct verb tense.

Phase 3:   **Future tense**. Use "is going to . . ." form of verb to start. Later you can teach "will . . ." form (this is used less often in everyday language).

For SD1 and SD2 use the card set that shows three different phases of action. For example: 1) Person looking at a banana; 2) Person peeling a banana; 3) Banana peel laying on table in front of a person.

SD1a: Point to picture one. "What is [person] going to do?"

R1a: "[person] is going to . . ."

SD1b: Point to picture two. "What is [person] doing?"

R1b: "[person] is _____ing."

SD1c: Point to picture two. "What did [person] do?"

R1c: "[person] _____ed."

SD2:   Random rotation of past, present and future tense. Show card. "Tell me about the picture."

R2:   Student responds with sentence in correct verb tense.

SD3a: Tell Student to perform action. Delay him in starting action. "What are you going to do?"

R3a: "I am going to . . ."

SD3b: Release Student to perform action. As he is performing action, ask "What are you doing?"

R3b: "I am _____ing."

SD3c: Pause after action is completed. "What did you do?"

R3c: "I _____ed."

SD4:   Random rotation of past, present and future tense with Student performing the action. This is done by randomly omitting questions for step a) and/or b) with SD3 above, so that the order of questions is not predictable.

R4:   Student responds with a sentence in correct verb tense.

SD5a: Have Student tell a character to perform an action ("Tell Big Bird to jump"). Delay making the character perform the action. "What is [character] going to do?"

R5a: "[character] is going to . . ."

SD5b: Have the character perform the action. As it is performing the action, ask "what is [character] doing?"

R5b: "[character] is _____ing."

SD5c: Pause after the action is completed. "What did [character] do?"

R5c: "[character] _____ed."

SD6:   Random rotation of past, present and future tense with a character performing an action. This is done by randomly omitting questions for step a) and/or b) with SD5 above, so that the order of questions is not predictable.

R6:   Student responds with a sentence in correct verb tense.

Cross-Refer: Recall
Expanding Language I

Plurals

Objectives: 1.   Increase correct use of grammar

                       2.   Establish awareness of quantity

Procedure: Student will be presented with a choice of items to make a correct match of singular *vs.* plural with corresponding language.

Prompts: Use physical guidance, demonstration, verbal, pointing or position prompt. Gradually fade the prompts until Student performs independently.

Entry criter: Completion of big vs. small and more vs. less.

Mastery crit: Student performs a response nine out of ten times correctly with no prompting. This should be repeated with at least one additional teacher.

Phase 1:   **Receptive discrimination.** Present two piles of an item (*e.g.*, blocks). One pile has a single block. The other has two or more blocks. Tell Student to "touch block" *vs.* "touch blocks." This should be done with various 3-D objects as well as with pictures.

Phase 2:   **Expressive labeling.** Show Student a pile that has one or more of an item in it (*e.g.*, cars). Ask, "what is it?" He should respond "car" or "cars."

Phase 3:   **Expressive verbs.** Show Student pictures of an action and ask a question that requires using the correct form of verb. Provide the correct noun in the question.

                    What does Daddy eat for breakfast?
                    What are the boys doing?
                    Where do the children live?

Phase 4:   **Expanding grammar.** Once Student has the basic idea of singular *vs.* plural, teach him now to say complete sentences using a variety of phrases.

                    What is this? It's a car.
                    What are these? These are cars.

What do you see? I see a car.
What do you see? I see some cars.

Phase 5:   **Teach student to match verb form with singular *vs.* plural subject**.
Show pictures of persons carrying out an action and ask, "What is happening?"

The boy is swimming.
The boys are swimming.
Mommy is waving.
Mommy and Daddy are waving.

Phase 6:   **Writing**. Student fills in the blanks in sentences, using singular *vs.* plural for nouns and verbs.

Cross-Refer: Describing
Verb tenses

"I Don't Know"

Objectives:

1. Provide a means of answering a question when Student does not know the answer

2. "I don't know" will become the precursor to seeking information (*e.g.*, "What is it?")

3. Reduce echolalia (echolalia is often exhibited when an answer is unknown)

4. Provide the teacher with a method to identify knowledge deficits

5. Reduce guessing

Procedure: The goal is for Student to say "I don't know" when asked the name or function of an unknown object. Ask him to identify a variety of objects that he knows as well as objects that he does not know. Prompt him to state "I don't know" when asked to label unknown objects. Eventually, he should be taught to ask the name of the object (*i.e.*, "What is it?").

Phase 1: **Student is asked to identify a variety of objects that he knows as well as objects that he does not know.** Student should then be prompted to state "I don't know" when asked to label unknown objects. If he tries to come up with a name and it is incorrect, say "don't guess."

When "I don't know" is established, randomize trials with known objects. It is important to **provide reinforcement for labeling known objects** as well as saying "I don't know." Otherwise he may label even known objects as "I don't know."

a. SD: What is it? R: I don't know.

b. SD: Who is it? R: I don't know.

c. SD: Where is it? R: I don't know.

Phase 2:   **Student should be taught to ask someone the name of the object by inquiring.** Show him a series of items or pictures. Have him label the items that are known. For those he does not know, he should ask the appropriate question:

a.   What is it?

b.   Who is it?

c.   Where is it?

Phase 3:   **Ask Student informational questions to which he does not know the answer.**
(*e.g.*, "What are you going to have for dinner?"). Initially the questions should be relevant to him. Eventually, more general information questions should be asked. **IT IS IMPORTANT THAT THE INFORMATION BE FUNCTIONAL, MOTIVATING AND AGE APPROPRIATE.**

Phase 4:   **Vary the language used.** Ask Student a question that does not make sense and teach him to respond "I don't understand"; "What did you say?"; "Can you say that again?"or other commonly used phrases.

Cross-Refer: Assertiveness
Expressive Labels
Observational Learning

Conversation — Intermediate

Objectives:

1. Develop a means for social interaction

2. Expand length of utterance

3. Teach conversational strategies

4 . Increase acceptance by peers

5. Teach Student to attend and respond to verbal input of others.

Procedure:

The goal is for Student to learn conversational skills. Initially, he will learn to answer simple questions. Gradually, questions will require increased language and progress to more complex conversational skills.

Questions should be age-appropriate, and the types of questions that peers would ask. Moreover, the responses should also be age-appropriate. In response to "How are you?," instead of responding "Fine, thank you," a more typical answer would be "Okay" or "All right." Therefore, it is essential to observe Student's peers to identify conversational objectives.

Phase 1:

Answering open-ended questions (rote memory)
a. What's your name? (B: 2-0)
b. How old are you? (B: 3-0)
c. Who do you love/Who loves you? How much?
d. Where do you go to school?
e. Who is your teacher?
f. What kids are in your class?
g. Where do you live? (B: 4-0)
h. What is your phone number?
i. What color is your house?
j. What is your cat's name?
k. Where does Grandma live?
l. What color is your hair?

Phase 2:   **Answering subjective questions**
-     a.   What do you like to eat?
-     b.   What do you like to drink?
-     c.   What color do you like?
-     d.   What's your favorite TV show?
-     e.   What do you like to do at school?
-     f.   What do you like to do after school?

Phase 3:   **Answering Yes/No Questions**
-     a.   Do you have a brother?
-     b.   Do you have a sister?
-     c.   Do you have any pets?
-     d.   Do you like power rangers?
-     e.   Do you like to play soccer?
-     f.   Are you a boy/girl?
-     g.   Do you wear glasses?
-     h.   Is mommy's car blue/white/etc?
-     i.   Do you like pizza?
-     j.   Do you have a bike?

Phase 4:   **Conversational questions** (answers may change)
-     a.   Where is (person)?
-     b.   How is the weather?
-     c.   What did you eat for breakfast?
-     d.   What are you doing?

Phase 5:   **Answering multiple choice questions**
-     a.   Do you want strawberry or chocolate ice cream?
-     b.   Is that dog big or little?

Phase 6:   **Asking Reciprocal Questions**
-     a.   How are you? ("Fine, how are you?")
-     b.   What's your name? ("Student. What's your name?")
-     c.   How old are you? ("Five. How old are you?")
-     d.   What did you have for dinner last night? ("Spaghetti and salad. What did you have for dinner?")

Phase 7:   **Statement/Statement**
-     a.   I'm wearing a blue shirt. ("I'm wearing a red shirt.")
-     b.   I'm holding a pencil. ("I'm holding an eraser.")
-     c.   My name is Ron. ("My name is Student.")
-     d.   I like to play baseball. ("I like basketball.")

Phase 8: **Statement/Question**

    a.   I went to the movies ("What did you see?")

    b.   I have a dog ("What's his name?")

    c.   I had a fun weekend ("What did you do?")

    d.   Basketball is my favorite sport. ("What's your favorite team?)

Phase 9: **Statement/Negative Statement**

    a.   I like hamburgers. (I don't like hamburgers. I like hot dogs better.)

    b.   I like swimming in the ocean. (I don't like the ocean. The waves are too big.)

Phase 10: **Statement/Statement/Question**

    a.   I like ice cream. ("I love cake and ice cream, do you like cake too?")

    b.   I hate doing the laundry. ("I hate taking out the trash. How about you?")

    c.   I like Friends. ("I like the Simpsons. Do you watch that show?")

    d.   I'm going to the movies. ("Me too. What are you seeing?")

    e.   For familiar story, movie etc., asks, "Did you like the part where . . ."

Asking Questions

Objectives:	1. Increase Student's awareness of his environment and actions that people are performing
	2. Provide a means of obtaining information
Procedure:	A situation is set up to induce Student to ask a question. There will be some type of reward for asking questions. The goal is to have him initiate questions in response to naturally occurring events.
Prompts:	Use verbal or gestural prompt. Gradually fade the prompts until Student performs independently.
Mastery crit:	Student asks an appropriate question four out of five times with no prompting. This should be repeated with at least one additional teacher.
Phase 1:	a) **What is it/What's that?** Arrange for some unfamiliar object to be displayed in obvious view. Initially, make it a specific location and on each trial you should pass by the location. Prompt Student to ask appropriate question. Do repeated trials as necessary. After he catches on, begin to vary the location and space out the trials.
	b) **Put out a few objects (some known, some unknown) and ask, "What do you see?"** Student names items and asks "What is it?" when he comes to an unknown item.
Phase 2:	**Who is it?** Present photos of people, some that are known, and some that are unknown. Start by asking "Who is it?," but fade out the question and turn it into commenting. For example, as you present a picture say, "Oh, look at this!" If it is an unfamiliar person, student should say, "Who is it?"
Phase 3:	a) **Where is it?** Have a favorite item hidden in the room. Tell Student, "There's a [object] in the room." When he asks where, show him or give verbal directions on how to find it. Another variation is to say "Mom knows," and have him go ask her (or another person).
	b) **Set Student up to do an activity** (*e.g.*, painting), but leave out one

important part (*e.g.*, brush). Student should ask, "Where's the [brush]?"

c) Put some items on a table. Ask Student to bring you an item. If the requested item is on the table, he should bring it. If not, he should ask, "Where's the [item]?"

Phase 4:   **What are you doing?** With great drama, the teacher turns away from Student, looking back over her shoulder. Student is prompted to ask, "What are you doing?"

Blowing up a balloon
Drawing a picture
Winding up a toy
Doing a puzzle
Getting ready to tickle you

Phase 5:   **What's in there?** The teacher puts something in a box and shakes it enticingly in front of Student. Generalize this by putting a conspicuous container in the environment and give an indication that there is something inside.

Phase 6:   **Where are you going?** The teacher gets up and leaves the room. Do this in a manner that catches Student's attention. Prompt him to ask, "Where are you going?" The teacher gives an interesting answer and invites him to come along to:

The kitchen (to get a drink)
Get bubbles
Get a snack
Swing outside, jump on trampoline, etc.

Phase 7:   **Who has it?** Tell Student, "Someone has the [object]."

Phase 8:   **What's wrong?** The teacher sits by Student and cries or sighs heavily.

I broke my pencil
There's no one to tickle or play with me (then grab him and start playing)
I need help (with a simple task he enjoys)
I miss you (give me a big hug!)
My puppet fell asleep (have him wake it up)

**Additional
Questions:**

Where's the box?
Where's mom?
What time is it?
Can I do that/Can I play/Can I have a turn?
Who's here? (someone knocks on door, walks up steps, etc.)
How did you do that?
What should I do?
How should I do it?

Cross-Refer:

I Don't Know
Expanding Language I
Conversation

Sequencing

Objectives: 1.   Increase familiarity with the order of events in everyday life

2.   Develop abstract reasoning and problem solving skills

3.   Establish understanding of cause and effect

4.   Increase social and environmental awareness

5.   Expand use of expressive language

6.   Develop story telling skills

Procedure: Use cards with pictures of scenes, or use number and letter flashcards. Start with sequences that have three scenes. Select pictures that clearly the progression of activity. Write a one sentence description of the scene on the back of the card for reference by all teachers. The sentence should be different for each card and should capture what is unique about that scene. The goal is for Student to put the cards in order. Use left to right positioning on the table in front of him. After the cards are in order, have Student tell you the story. The purpose of this is to introduce him to the process of telling a simple story using pictures as a prompt.

Amusing and interesting sequences will maintain motivation. You can make up your own cards by taking pictures from a story or making photographs of Student and familiar persons. This will promote generalization and make the skill more functional.

Entry criter: Sorting is a prerequisite.

Mastery crit: Student performs a response four out of five times correctly with no prompting. This should be repeated with at least one additional teacher.

Phase 1:   **Three-card sequence**. Present card one and prompt Student to describe the picture. Tell him this card is first and show him where to place the card on the table and have him put the card on the table. Present card two and do the same, telling him that this card is next. Repeat for card three, saying this is last. Review sequence as many times as needed until Student is correctly describing the scene and putting the card on the table with no prompt.

At this point, begin a backward chaining procedure. Present the first card, have Student describe the picture and tell him to "Put this in order." Have him put the card on the left side of the table. Present the two remaining cards together in a random pile away from the first card. Ask, "What comes next?" Guide him as needed to select the second card and put it down to the right of the first card. Then have him put down the third card at the end of the row. Finally, say to him, "Tell me the story."

Once Student is correctly placing cards two and three, start giving him all three cards together in a random pile. Tell him, "put these in order." When the cards are in place, have him tell you the story.

NOTE: Phases 2 and 3 may be easier for some students to learn first.

Phase 2:   **Ordering three alphabet cards** (*e.g.*, A - B - C)

Phase 3:   **Ordering three number cards** (*e.g.*, 1 - 2 - 3)

Phase 4:   **Four-card sequence**. Use the above procedure to teach the ordering of four cards using backward chaining. Step 1 is ordering cards 3 and 4, after cards 1 and 2 are already on the table. Step 2 is ordering cards 2, 3, and 4. Step 3 is ordering all four cards.

Phase 5:   **What happens next?** Once Student is familiar with describing the sequence, point to the empty space to the right of the last picture and ask, "What happens next?" Give verbal prompt to elicit a plausible answer.

Phase 6:   **Five- and six-card picture sequence**

Phase 7:   **Ordering four to six alphabet cards**

Phase 8:   **Ordering four to six number cards**

Cross-Refer: Quantitative Skills
                Cause & Effect

First/Last

Objectives: 1. Incorporate sequencing into Student's use of language

2. Increase attention to the temporal relationship between events

3. Improve recall

Procedure: Student is instructed to perform a response. He is then quizzed about what happened first or last.

Prompts: Use physical guidance, demonstration, verbal, pointing or temporal prompt. Gradually fade the prompts until Student performs independently.

Entry criter: Student should be able to arrange items in simple sequences and should have mastered multiple step (at least two) receptive instructions.

Mastery crit: Student performs a response nine out of ten times correctly with no prompting with two choices, eight out of ten times with three or more choices. This should be repeated with at least one additional teacher.

Phase 1: **Have Student arrange three or more sequence cards that he has previously learned in correct order.**

SD1: "Touch first"
R1: Student touches the card that is first in the sequence (always on the left).

SD2: "Touch last"
R2: Student touches the card that is last in the sequence.

SD3: Random rotation of SD1 *vs.* SD2

This can also be done with numbers and letters.

Phase 2: **Arrange a number of animals (or other characters, people, etc.) all in a line facing in the same direction.**

Example: lined up to get on a bus

SD1:	"Who is first?"
R1:	Student points to the figure that is first in the line.

SD2:	"Who is last?"
R2:	Student points to the figure that is last in the sequence.

SD3:	Random rotation of SD1 vs. SD2

SD4:	Have the line going in various directions so that Student is not dependent on left vs. right location.

Phase 3a:	**Put out two items. Tell him, "touch [item one] first."** After he touches it, then tell him "touch [item two] last." The set of objects should be varied on every trial. Using the words "first" and "last" in the instruction is a prompt that will be faded later.

Please note that you have previously taught Student to complete two or three-step instructions in correct order in the Receptive Instructions program. In that program, even if you included the words "first" and "last" in the instructions, this would not be sufficient to teach the concept of first vs. last. The reason is because the order of first vs. last is never randomized in the Receptive Instructions program. In the First vs. Last program, the emphasis is on Student **RECALLING** the order in which he did various actions and therefore first and last can be randomized.

SD1:	"What did you touch last?"
R1:	Student names the item that he touched last.

Phase 3b:	SD2a:	"What did you touch last?"
R2a:	Student names the item that he touched last.
SD2b:	"What did you touch first?"
R2b:	Student names the item that he touched first.

Phase 3c:	SD3:	"What did you touch first?"
R3:	Student names the item that he touched first.

Phase 3d:	Random alternation between first and last.

Phase 3e:	Drop the words "first" and "last" when you are telling him to touch the items in the setup. Once he is good at SD5 with two items then put out three items. Giving him one instruction at a time, have him touch each of the three items.

Phase 3f: Random rotation of "What did you touch first?" *vs.* "What did you touch last?" in a field of three.

Phase 4a: **Actions in environment**. Tell Student to do [action one]. After he does that, tell him to do [action two]. The set of actions should be varied on every trial. If necessary, the words "first" and "last" can be used in the instruction and faded later.

SD1:   "What did you do last?"
R1:   Student names the action that he did last.

Phase 4b: SD2a: "What did you do last?"
R2a: Student names the action that he did last.
SD2b: "What did you do first?"
R2b: Student names the action that he did first.

Phase 4c: SD3:   "What did you do first?"
R3:   Student names the action that he did first.

Phase 4d: Random alternation between first and last.

Phase 4e: Once he is good at Phase 4e with two actions then have him perform three actions, giving one instruction at a time. Randomly rotate "What did you do first?" *vs.* "What did you do last?" in a field of three.

Cross-Refer: Sequencing
Before/After
Receptive Instructions
Recall
Verb Tense

Before/After

Objectives:

1. Incorporate sequencing into Student's use of language

2. Increase attention to the temporal relationship between events

3. Improve recall

4. Establish ability to carry out complex instructions

Prompts: Use physical guidance, demonstration, verbal, pointing or position prompt. Gradually fade the prompts until Student performs independently.

Entry criter: Student should have mastered First/Last and Sequencing. Most children who are ready for this program will also have started using verb tenses correctly.

Mastery crit: Student performs a response nine out of ten times correctly with no prompting with two choices, eight out of ten times with three or more choices. This should be repeated with at least one additional teacher.

Phase 1: **Identifies which item comes before or after a specific point in a series.**

a) Numbers. Have Student put several numbers in order (*e.g.*, 1-5). He should line them up in a row on the table from least to most. Tell him to point to a reference number (*e.g.*, 3). Put a marker on that number. Then ask him to tell you which number comes before or after the reference number (*e.g.*, "What comes before 3?").

b) Letters of alphabet. Follow same procedure as 1a), except use letters of the alphabet.

c) Days of week. Use a strip that lists the days of the week in order. Follow same procedure as 1a).

d) Picture sequence. Have Student line up scenes in a row on the table. Ask him questions about what happened before or after a certain event in the sequence (*e.g.*, Q: "What did the boy do before he ate the banana?" A: "He peeled it." Q: "What did he do after he ate it?" A: He threw it away).

Phase 2:   **Student carries out a series of responses and answers questions about what he did before or after one of those responses**. Teacher should have him do at least three responses. The reference item should be something other than the first or last step. If it is a three-step chain, ask about the response before or after the middle step. Example:

T: "Close the door."
S: Closes door.
T: "Clap your hands."
S: Claps hands.
T: "Kick the ball."
S: Kicks ball.
T: "What did you do before you clapped?"
S: "I closed the door"
T: "What did you do after you clapped?"
S: "I kicked the ball."

Phase 3:   **Student carries out instructions that include the word before or after**

Cross-Refer: Recall
First/Last
Sequencing

Stories

Objectives:

1. Expose Student to books, which are an important source of future learning

2. Expand range of experience

3. Provide stimulus material for development of language

4. Establish additional reinforcers

5. Establish additional leisure activity

Procedure: Have Student listen to stories that you read to him. Use books (*e.g.*, bugs, dinosaurs, Sesame Street, etc.) that he would like and that tell an interesting story and have good pictures. In the beginning, try using books that have flaps to open, or push buttons that make sounds. Monitor Student's behavior closely to ensure that he is listening to the story. Keep him actively involved in the activity by pointing to things in the pictures, answering questions, and turning the pages. Do not let him turn the page before it is time. Try to ask a question on every page or after every two to four sentences. Incorporate concepts that you are working on in other programs (*e.g.*, naming objects, colors, prepositions, cause & effect, emotions, functions).

Phase 1: **Increase the amount of time Student spends listening to a story**. Use generous reinforcement to maintain a high level of interest.

Phase 2: **Have him receptively identify concepts that have been taught in other programs.**

Phase 3: **Have him expressively label concepts that have been taught in other programs.**

Phase 4: **Guess what happens next.**

Phase 5: **Explain why something happened.**

Phase 6: **Encourage the use of books as an independent activity.**

Phase 7: **Have Student summarize a story you or he has read**. Include listing characters, telling the main points, how it ended, and how he liked the story.

Phase 8: **Have Student make up a story, draw the illustrations, and create a book**. This may be done one page at a time over a series of days.

Phase 9: **Story weaving**. The teacher and Student take turns adding a sentences to a story that begins with, "Once upon a time. . ." Prompt him with partial sentences as needed (*e.g.*, "There was a boy named . . ."; "He lived . . ."; "One day . . .").

Phase 10: **Telling a complete story**. Have Student make up a complete story. At first, prompt him to include three components, the beginning, middle, and end. Gradually increase the complexity of stories being told. To get him accustomed to the process, you can start with retelling familiar stories that he has heard numerous times.

Cause And Effect

Objectives:	1.	Learn temporal relationships
	2.	Learn sequence of events
	3.	Predict what occurs after events
	4.	Identify repercussions of behaviors
	5.	Learn to make inference from events
	6.	Develop abstract reasoning
	7.	Learns what to do in situations (*i.e.*, problem solving skills)

Procedure: Initially, Student will observe events happening and will be asked to identify cause and effect. Later he will be shown a series of events depicted in pictures. Student will be taught to identify the order of events. Eventually he will make inferences regarding events.

Phase 1:   **Demonstrate or role-play an action with an obvious outcome**. Ask Student to explain why the outcome happened.

SIMPLE

Cause	Effect
turn light off	room is dark
take away toy	person cries
object is dropped	object is on floor
tickle person	person laughs
"I'm hungry"	eat
"I'm thirsty"	drink
(yawn) "I'm tired"	sleep
hurt self	cry
give something	person happy/smiles
scrape knee	bleed
towel in water	towel now wet
drop egg	egg broken
drink	glass empty
eat	food gone

go swimming	all wet
sprayed by squirt	gun dripping
took a shower	hair wet
wind up	toy moves
turn on radio	music plays
turn on VCR	video plays
microwave food	HOT!! HOT!!
flush toilet	bye bye poo/tissue
play in mud	hands dirty
wash with soap	hands clean
BM accident	soiled pants
cut with knife	fruit is split
knock at door	dogs bark
telephone rings	adult answers phone

ADVANCED

Cause	Effect
insult delivered	person cries
child hits classmate	time out chair
child ill (*e.g.*, vomits)	go to nurse's office
ice cream left out	melts
toy train tracks come undone	derails
pants zipper undone	kids laugh
cleans plate	gets dessert
disobey mom	mom angry/scolds
throw ball in house	lamp broken

Generalize this concept to everyday events as they happen.

Example:
Teacher: Why did your crayons melt?
Student: Because I left them in the sun.
Teacher: Why did the sun melt the crayons?
Student: Because the sun is hot.

Phase 2:   **Show Student sequence cards in order, leaving out one card and have him describe the event that is missing.**

Phase 3:   **Show Student the cards in order and have him tell you what happened prior to the sequence.**

Phase 4:   **Show Student the cards in order and have him tell you what is likely to happen after the last picture.**

Phase 5.   **Show Student a picture and ask a question that requires an inference** (*e.g.*, "Why is the girl crying?"; "Why is the boy eating?"; "Why is the lady packing a suitcase?" etc.)

Phase 6:   **Ask questions as described above while reading stories.** Fade out reliance on a picture as a visual cue.

Phase 7:   **Intra-verbal.** Ask "why" questions that draw on general knowledge and information Student has learned. (*e.g.*, "Why do we eat?"; "Why do birds have wings?")

Cross-Refer: Sequencing
                      What's Missing?

Comprehension I

Objectives: 1.   Establish discrimination of wh- questions

2.   Increase attention to visual input.

3.   Improve understanding of information that is received through listening or reading

Procedure: Ask Student a question which requires utilization of information that he has just received (read or heard), or can be answered by looking around the environment or in a picture.

Prompts: Use physical guidance, demonstration, verbal, pointing or position prompt. Gradually fade the prompts until Student performs independently.

Mastery crit: Student performs a response nine out of ten times correctly. This should be repeated with at least one additional teacher.

Phase 1:   **What?**

Phase 2:   **What color?**

Phase 3:   **What *vs.* What color?**

Phase 4:   **Who?**

Phase 5:   **Who *vs.* What?**

Phase 6:   **(What) doing?**

Phase 7:   **Who *vs.* What *vs.* (What) doing?**

Phase 8:   **Where?**

Phase 9:   **Who *vs.* What *vs.* (What) doing *vs.* Where?**

Phase 10:   **Which?**

Phase 11:   **Who *vs.* What *vs.* (What) doing *vs.* Where *vs.* Which?**

Phase 12:   **How?**

Phase 13:   **Who *vs.* What *vs.* (What) doing *vs.* Where *vs.* Which *vs.* How?**

Comprehension II

Objectives:
1. Enable Student to answer common questions about information he has acquired

2. Increase his attention to auditory and visual input

3. Establish discrimination of wh- questions

Procedure: Ask Student a question which requires utilization of general knowledge and information that has been previously acquired.

Prompts: Use physical guidance, demonstration, verbal, pointing or position prompt. Gradually fade the prompts until Student performs independently.

Mastery crit: Student performs a response nine out of ten times correctly. This should be repeated with at least one additional teacher.

Phase 1: Who?

Phase 2: Who *vs.* (What) doing?

Phase 3: Who *vs.* (What) doing *vs.* What *vs.* What color?

Phase 4: Who *vs.* (What) doing *vs.* What *vs.* What color *vs.* Where?

Phase 5: Who *vs.* (What) doing *vs.* What *vs.* What color *vs.* Where *vs.* When?

Phase 6: Who *vs.* (What) doing *vs.* What *vs.* What color *vs.* Where *vs.* When *vs.* Which?

Phase 7: Who *vs.* (What) doing *vs.* What *vs.* What color *vs.* Where *vs.* When *vs.* Which *vs.* Why?

Phase 8: Who *vs.* (What) doing *vs.* What *vs.* What color *vs.* Where *vs.* When *vs.* Which *vs.* Why *vs.* How?

Peer Interaction

Objectives:

1. Establish and increase responses to peer initiation of communication, play, and cooperative activities

2. Establish and increase initiation of these activities with peers

3. Facilitate language—children's language is often enhanced as a result of observing and engaging with peers

4. Increasing observational skills

5. Serves as a comparison standard for Student's social, language and play skills

Procedure:

These are activities that are suitable for teaching and promoting interaction with peers.

In preparation for the peer sessions, appropriate play skills should be identified and taught in one-on-one discrete trial sessions. Selection of play skills should be based upon which play skills will facilitate social integration, as well as which play would Student enjoy most. Play must be age-appropriate.

When Student has learned a few play skills begin the peer interaction with brief sessions. For example, arrange for the peer to come over for 30 minutes. The first couple of sessions should be aimed at making the experience highly reinforcing for both Student and the peer. This may mean no formal teaching until both children are hooked on the reinforcers (*e.g.*, baking chocolate chip cookies, making Kool-Aid, playing with a great toy, swimming in the pool, etc.). In particular, the peer should leave eagerly looking forward to the next visit.

The second phase consists of implementing no more than three "trials" of about three minutes duration each. However, the peer should not be able to tell that you are doing "therapy." The adult's role should be as informal as possible. Do not overly structure the activity, but have in mind a script that you can fall back on if the play stalls or goes in a wrong direction. The script is really a guideline for the therapist to follow if prompting is necessary. Select activities that are mutually enjoyable and interactive. During each trial, do a different activity. Each activity should be one that Student is already familiar with from previous training. For each activity, you should develop specific goals for behaviors you want to occur. For example, language to use, eye contact, turn taking, where to be, what to do. Naturally, staff should understand age-appropriate conversation, behavior and interactions so that they facilitate age-appropriate interactions. Sometimes staff views play with an adult eye and therefore create adult play behavior.

Be sure to reinforce the peer for cooperative behavior. Prompt the peer if necessary to ask questions and give directives to Student. Make sure Student responds to the peer. Don't let the peer do things for Student. If Student takes a toy from the peer, have him give it back. If the peer asks the adult a question, have the peer ask Student. The adult should not become the focus of the peer's interactions.

In between the formal trials, let the children do whatever they want, including playing separately. Be flexible with the time guidelines. You may be able to adjust them very quickly. Spontaneous behavior should always take precedence over the script. Never interrupt something positive that is happening. Do not be too quick to give directives or prompts so that there is ample opportunity for spontaneous behavior to occur.

Gradually lengthen the duration of the trials and the length of the overall play session.

Factors in Peer Selection: Peers that possess good social, play and communication skills are critical. Additionally, the peer should be someone who will be persistent or even bossy, but will take direction well from an adult. In the beginning, this may work better with a peer who is a little older.

Prompts: Use physical guidance, demonstration, verbal, or gestural prompt. Gradually fade the prompts until Student performs independently.

Entry criter: Disruptive behaviors should be minimal so as not to alienate the peer.

Mastery crit: Student performs and remains on task 80 percent of the time and responds to 80 percent of opportunities for interaction.

Examples:

Highly Structured - Indoors
Send wind-up car back and forth
Table games
Play catch
Build something cooperatively
Put puzzle together
Matchbox cars/train set/hot wheels/race set

Cooperative Tasks (Labeling; Expanding Language I; Describing; Requesting; Taking turns; Assisting each other):
Food preparation
Building something

Creative Activities
Make something with Playdoh (each person does part of it to contribute to the final product).
Work on projects in parallel and show each other the end product (*e.g.*, art). Student needs to ask for things and respond to requests from peer (*e.g.*, crayons).

Outdoors
Ride on seesaw
Take turns going down slide
Roll ball down slide to other person
Take turns riding and pulling wagon
Sand box play

Language-based
Have peer be teacher for teaching program (*e.g.*, Nonverbal Imitation)
Have Student be teacher for peer (*e.g.*, Nonverbal Imitation)
Language programs: statement-statement; reciprocal questions
Conversation
Story time

Movement Games
Follow-the-leader
Ring-around-the-rosie
Hide and seek
Musical chairs; freeze dancing
Tag
Hunting for bugs
Cops and Robbers; Cowboys and Indians; etc.

Imaginative Play With Props

Act out scripts: "Thomas the train"; Aladdin
Build a "fort" or "tent"
Play with play sets: Legos; castles; doll house
Play "Doctor"
Dress up
Pushing chair cubes around pretending to drive
Pretend store; shopping trip; ice cream parlor, etc.

Conversation – Advanced

Objectives:

1. Provide a basis and structure for conversations

2. Become more aware of peers

3. Provide a means for social interaction, making and sustaining friendships

4. To get along with others in school, work and leisure settings

5. Learn information about interests of peers

6. Expand Student's horizons to include enjoyment of a broader range of experience

Procedure:

The program involves initially providing Student with rote conversational skills. Eventually, these conversations will become more natural.

Identify areas that may be of interest to him. More important, perhaps, is to identify topics that may facilitate a peer's interest in conversing with him.

Topic Examples

1. Toys
2. Interests
3. School
4. What happened last weekend
5. What is going to happen next weekend
6. Describing what is currently happening
7. Significant occurrences
8. TV shows
9. Favorite characters
10. Movies/Videos
11. Music
12. Computer Games
13. Sports
14. Extra Curricular Activities

15.   Vacations
16.   Current Events
17.   Places to Go
18.   Clothes Shopping
19.   Celebrities
20.   Friends
21.   Opposite Sex

TOPICS ARE BASED UPON AGE, DEVELOPMENTAL LEVEL, LANGUAGE & INTERESTS

Phase 1: **Tell *vs.* Ask**. Follow basic discrimination training procedure. Teach Student to respond correctly to the two instructions. Example: "Tell Mom about lunch" *vs.* "Ask Mom about lunch."

Phase 2: **Appropriate nonverbal conversational skills** (*e.g.*, proximity, eye contact, smiling, nodding, etc.). Engage in conversation with Student and reinforce him for displaying appropriate nonverbal behavior. Prompt as needed.

Phase 3: **Conversational manners** (*e.g.*, listening, waiting to interject, how to stay on topic, how to make a transition, etc.). Engage in conversation with Student and reinforce him for displaying appropriate conversational manners. Prompt as needed.

Phase 4: **Conversational Topics.** Generate a list of topics that would be appropriate for Student to include in conversation with peers and familiar adults. For each topic, have him list items that he could mention in a conversation about the topic.

Phase 5: **Teach Student to respond to simple questions regarding the selected topic** (*e.g.*, What, where, when, etc.)

Phase 6: **Teach Student to reciprocate statements regarding the selected topic**. See Phase 7 of Conversation-Intermediate.

Phase 7: **Teach Student to ask questions**. Start this when he is able to discriminate among all the different "WH" questions. To prompt this, tell him to ask peer a question and then show an index card with one of the "WH" words written on it (*e.g.*, "WHAT"). For example, Student may start with "WHAT did you do last night?" When he gets the answer, prompt for a follow-up question (*e.g.*, "WHO"). He should ask something like, "Who went with you?"

Phase 8.   **Teach him how to appropriately interject information.** "Do you know what I did today?" "Guess what."

Phase 9.   **Teach him how to identify interests of other persons.** Start with having him query various persons and make a list of things they find interesting *vs.* boring. Later, present various topics to him and have him discriminate between topics that a certain person would or would not find interesting.

Phase 10:   **Have him initiate a conversation with someone by telling them something interesting.** He should start out with a statement like, "Guess what . . ." or "Hey, Joe . . ." or "Wanna know . . .?" Topics could include such things as a current event or something he did recently.

Phase 11:   **Teach him to identify when peers become disinterested in conversation.** Use role-playing and video tape examples to practice this skill. Then set up real life examples. Reinforce him for correctly reading cues of the other person. For example, smiling and eye contact indicate interest. Looking away, fidgeting, or checking time indicate disinterest.

Phase 12:   **Teach him how to recall previous conversations within current conversation.** This requires carrying on a conversation about a memorable topic and then testing Student at a subsequent time to see what he can recall about that conversation. Initially, the delay between performance and recall may need to be brief. To aid in recall, you can also use anchors such as referring to the location where the conversation took place.

Conversation Checklist

MARK 1-5 (5 IS BEST).

____ Appropriate distance (not too close, not too far)

____ Maintains appropriate eye contact

____ No inappropriate touching

____ Acknowledges statements of other person (nod, smile, etc.)

____ No interrupting or cutting off

____ Listens to what other person says

____ Stays on topic

____ No abrupt shifts of topic; no jumping around on topics

____ Brings up new topic gracefully

____ Leaves old topic behind when conversation has changed topic

____ Is attuned to what other person finds interesting

____ No rude comments about other people's appearance or behavior

____ Allows other person to have turns to talk

____ Does not talk over other person

____ Ends conversation gracefully

____ Appropriate volume

Social Awareness

A. Learning from modeling prompt

   1. verbal
   2. visual

B. Greetings

   1. respond
   2. initiate

C. Sharing and Cooperation

   1. Taking turns
   2. Losing graciously

D. Identify which person in group:

   1. holds a particular object
   2. has certain attribute (hair color, blue sweater, etc.)
   3. is performing a particular action
   4. said a particular phrase
   5. other information (*e.g.*, likes, dislikes)

E. Attends to verbal input in group setting

   1. Remains in designated place during group activity
   2. Performs action in unison with group
   3. Sings song in unison with group
   4. Looks toward speaker
   5. Responds to group questions
   6. Follows group directions
   7. Someone says, "I see X, Y, Z." Teacher asks, "What does [person] see?"
   8. Someone tells about something they did; teacher then asks, "What did [person] do?" or "Who [does action]?"
   9. Someone says, "I like to X, Y, Z." Teacher then asks, "What does [person] like to do?"

F.   Giving information to group/circle games

    1.   Tell me about yourself: "I have blue eyes . . ."
    2.   Describe another person
    3.   Statement/statement
    4.   Name item that belongs in category

G.   Seeks information

    1.   To facilitate Student asking questions to members of the group, ask him something he does not know about a person. Prompt him to say "I don't know", then prompt him to ask the person. Fade the prompts.

    2.   When he is asking questions reliably, change the instruction to "Ask [person] a question." At this point, he has to come up with the question on his own.

Observational Learning

Objectives:

1. Student learns to attend without direct instruction

2. Acquisition of concepts or information by listening and watching others

3. Learning through a more natural method of instruction, thereby facilitating inclusion into more natural educational settings

4. Develop social skills

5. Develop awareness and attending skills

6. Develop retention

7. Learning to wait his turn

8. Develop age appropriate social behavior (*e.g.*, becoming aware of hair styles, clothes, lunch boxes, interests, etc.)

Procedure:

The format involves asking questions of an accomplice (ideally a peer but perhaps initially another adult). Subsequently, ask Student the same question, and provide reinforcement for the correct response. Attempt to delay asking him the question, so as to facilitate attention. To increase difficulty, ask two or more persons questions with different answers, before giving Student a turn to answer. Then he must sort through a larger amount of information to come up with the correct answer to the question.

Gradually, the instructions and questions should become more complex. BE CAREFUL NOT TO OVERDO CUING TO PAY ATTENTION. YOU SHOULD FADE ANY ATTENTION PROMPTS AS QUICKLY AS POSSIBLE!!!

Prompts:

Use modeling as the main type of prompt. If a stronger prompt in needed, use direct verbal prompt or physical guidance. Gradually fade the prompt to a light touch and then a slight gesture.

Phase 1:   **Gets information about desired behavior from model..** When a motor response (*e.g.*, receptive instructions) needs to be prompted, let Student see a third person (*i.e.*, someone other than the teacher) model the action. For example, teacher says to Student, "Touch your nose." Student makes an incorrect response. Teacher gives feedback to Student and immediately turns to Suzy (who knows how to do it correctly) and asks her to do it. In the beginning, it may be necessary to specifically direct Student to watch Suzy, but the goal is for him to learn that he needs to watch Suzy without being told. By having someone other than the teacher demonstrate the correct response, Student learns the importance of observing what other people do.

a.   **Immediate:** Student is given an immediate opportunity to make the desired response

Example:
Teacher (to Johnny): "Touch your nose"
Johnny: Incorrect response
Teacher: "Uh-uh"
Teacher (to Suzy):   "Suzy, touch your nose"
Suzy: Responds correctly
Teacher (to Suzy);   "Nice job"
Teacher (to Johnny): "Touch your nose"

b.   **Delayed:** Student is provided with additional information or is distracted by a brief activity before having the opportunity to offer the response that was modeled for him.

Example:

Teacher (to Johnny): "Touch your nose"
Johnny: Incorrect response
Teacher: "Uh-uh"
Teacher (to Suzy):   "Suzy, touch your nose"
Suzy: Responds correctly
Teacher (to Suzy);   "Nice job"
Teacher (to Mary):   "Mary, stomp your feet"
Suzy: Responds correctly
Teacher (to Mary);   "Nice job"
Teacher (to Johnny): "Touch your nose"

Phase 2:   **Gets verbal information from model** (*e.g.*, expressive labels).

    a.   **Immediate:** Student is given an immediate opportunity to make the desired response

    b.   **Delayed:** Student is provided with additional information or is distracted by a brief activity before having the opportunity to offer the response which was modeled for him.

Phase 3:   **Choral Nonverbal Imitation.** Student performs nonverbal imitation responses in a group.

Phase 4:   **Do That.** Teacher points to another person and instructs Student to imitate that person.

Phase 5:   **Shell Game-watching.** Student observes an item being concealed beneath a container. Then that container is moved around in the field. He is asked to find the hidden item.

Phase 6:   **Choral Verbal Response.** Student makes a verbal response (*e.g.*, singing) in unison with a group.

Phase 7:   **I do/Not me!** In a circle game, ask questions that require Student to answer "I do" *vs.* "Not me" along with peers. Prompt him to give appropriate answers: I do! Not me! No way! Yuck!

    a.   Who wants . . .

        Who wants a tickle?
        Who wants a lemon?
        Who wants a hug?
        Who wants a pinch?
        Who wants a noogie?
        Who wants a snack?
        Who wants an onion?

    b.   Who has [item]?

Phase 8:   **In a group setting (*i.e.*, 2 or more) ask Student questions that require observation of group members** (*e.g.*, "who has a hat on their head," "who is holding a ball," "who is wearing blue jeans," etc.). Gradually, questions should require more keen observations. He should identify which person in group:

a.   holds a particular object: responds by pointing
b.   holds a particular object: responds by saying name of person
c.   has certain attribute (hair color, blue sweater, etc.)
d.   is performing a particular action

Phase 9:   **Every member of the group makes a statement about himself** (*e.g.*, "I like pizza," "I don't like cleaning my room," "I love the Dodgers," etc.). Student is then asked a question about the statement (*e.g.*, "Who likes pizza?" or "What does [person] like?").

a.   Who has (is holding) . . .
b.   Who likes . . .
c.   Who [did action]?
d.   Who went . . .

Phase 10:   **Information Acquisition-Verbal**. Have Student sit in circle with other persons. The objective is for Student to learn to listen while trials are occurring with other persons and wait for his turn. The teacher asks questions of other students and they are allowed to respond. Do not cue Student to attend, since the goal is for him to be able to observe events without being prompted. The teacher then asks Student a question about what was said.

The teacher should also have persons engage in general conversation. At various times after a person has said something, the teacher should turn to Student and ask what the person has just said.

a.   **Immediate:**

Example 1:
Teacher (to accomplice):	"Bobby, what time is it?"
Bobby:	"Three o'clock"
Teacher (to Student):	"Student, what time is it?"
Student:	Answers teacher's question.

Example 2:
Teacher (to accomplice):	"Heather, what did you have for breakfast?"
Heather:	"Cheerios"
Teacher (to Student):	"Student, what did Heather have for breakfast?"
Student:	Answers teacher's question.

      b.   **Delayed:** Student is provided with additional information or is distracted by a brief activity before having the opportunity to give a response.

Phase 11:   **Listens to incidental information.** For example, someone says to another person, "Hey, I brought some chocolate chip cookies for Student. He can have them whenever he wants."

Phase 12:   **Information Acquisition-Observation of activity.** Activity is staged or allowed to occur naturally. Do not cue Student to attend, since the goal is for him to be able to observe events without being prompted. Ask a question of Student about what happened (*e.g.*, "What did Ron do?" "Who bounced the ball?")

Phase 13:   **Detects incorrect answer or information.** Occasionally someone should give an incorrect answer and Student should catch it and correct the error.

Phase 14:   **Show accomplice a picture, without Student being able to see the picture.** Have accomplice describe what is in the picture.

      a.   Ask Student what accomplice saw. Student responds verbally.

      b.   Show two pictures to Student and ask which one the accomplice saw. Student points to correct picture. Eventually the pictures shown should be very similar and the dimension that the accomplice describes should be subtle (*e.g.*, a boy riding a bike with blue socks *vs.* a boy riding a bike with green socks).

Phase 15:   **Choral Group Instructions**

      a.   Addressed to entire group

      b.   Conditional (*e.g.*, "Everyone with red hair stand up," "Anyone who wants soda raise your hand," "If your name starts with 'H', wave goodbye," etc.)

Phase 16:   **Shell Game--deductive reasoning** Student observes another person make an incorrect guess about the location of a hidden item. He should use this information to narrow down the choices.

Phase 17:   **Drawing Inferences-Verbal**

                     Example 1:
                     Teacher: "Diane, what did you do this weekend?"
                     Diane: "I went to a carnival."
                     Teacher: "Student, do you think Diane had fun this weekend?"

                     Example 2:
                     Person 1: "I like pizza."
                     Person 2: "I like ice cream."
                     Teacher: "Student, who would go to Pizza Hut for lunch?"

Phase 18:   **Drawing Inferences-Observation of activity**. Have people demonstrate reactions to certain activities or items. Ask Student questions about these things (*e.g.*, "Would you like to try this?" "How did Marlene like that?" "Would Rick do that again?")

Phase 19:   **Ask Student to describe peer's interests**

Cross-Refer: Receptive Instructions
                     I Don't Know
                     Assertiveness
                     Expressive Labels

Socialization Skills

Objectives:	1.	Develop skills to facilitate social interaction
	2.	Reduce the disparity between Student and peers

Procedure: Initially Student will be taught prerequisite social skills in as natural a situation as possible. However, it may necessary to begin in a more structured teaching environment. Besides reducing possible distractions, it may help to avoid stigmatizing him due to inappropriate social behavior. Instructional procedures will include demonstration, role-playing and practice. Once critical skills are learned, he will practice and continue to develop skills in the most natural environment possible.

IT IS CRITICAL THAT SOCIAL SKILLS ARE AGE APPROPRIATE. THEREFORE, IT IS ADVISABLE TO OBSERVE PEERS IN ORDER TO IDENTIFY THEIR SOCIAL SKILLS.

General Strategy

1. Select target socialization skill.

2. Divide the skill into teachable parts.

3. Demonstrate the specific skill for Student.

4. Student should practice the skill until it is exhibited independently.

5. Set up a situation where he can practice the skill with accepting peers.

6. Fade the supervision while encouraging and reinforcing him for appropriate socialization.

Stages Of Social Development

1. Engages in simple game with others, such as rolling ball back and forth (B: 1-0)

2. Imitates actions of another child (B: 1-6)

3.   Watches other children play, and attempts to join briefly (B: 2-0)

4.   Plays alone, in presence of other children (B: 2-0)

5.   Watches others play and plays near them (B: 2-6)

6.   Plays simple group games (*e.g.*, Ring Around the Rosie) (B: 2-6)

7.   Begins to play with other children with adult supervision (B: 2-6)

8.   Begins to take turns (B: 3-0)

9.   Takes turns with assistance (B: 3-6)

10.   Forms temporary attachment to one playmate (B: 3-6)

11.   Can usually play cooperatively, but may need assistance (B: 3-6)

12.   Takes turns and shares, without supervision (B: 4-6)

13.   Plays cooperatively with up to two children for at least 15 minutes (B: 5-0)

14.   Has several friends, but one special friend (B: 5-0)

15.   Plays cooperatively in large group games (B: 5-6)

Examples:

Telling jokes
Seeking/Asking for attention appropriately
How to behave as a new person in a group
Refraining from odd behaviors (*e.g.*, funny voice)
What to do at a birthday party
Giving compliments
What to do when you see friends at the park

Interesting Places To Go:

Cub Scouts
Team Sports
Stores/Malls
Gymboree
Discovery Zone
Reading hour at library

Redirecting Inappropriate Behavior

That doesn't make sense
That sounds silly
Be cool/that's not cool
People will think that's weird
I don't get it
I don't want to talk about that
That's boring
Physical redirection (*e.g.*, have him put his hands in his pockets to suppress flapping)

What's Missing?

Objectives:

1. Develop awareness of environment

2. Develop memory

3. Games often involve "what's missing" concepts

Procedure:
A set of objects is placed in front of Student and he should scan them. Then he is told to close his eyes and one or more objects is removed. Student opens his eyes and the teacher asks, "What's missing?"

Phases

1. **Objects in front of Student**
   a. Teacher labels objects and then Student closes his eyes and object is removed. You can prompt this by covering up the object instead of removing it. Teacher asks, "What's missing?" Start with three objects.
   b. Student labels objects instead of teacher
   c. Student scans the field, instead of labeling objects

   SLOWLY INCREASE THE NUMBER OF OBJECTS.
   EVENTUALLY REMOVE MULTIPLE OBJECTS

2. **Pictures**. Put out a number of pictures in front of Student. Take one away and have him tell you which one is missing. This can also be done by drawing pictures on a dry erase board or chalkboard. The teacher or Student draws several pictures. Then he closes his eyes and one or more is erased.

3. **Objects in the environment** (*e.g.*, chair, plant, picture)

4. **"What's Different?"** Instead of removing objects just change them (*e.g.*, turn a table upside down) and ask "What's different?").

5. **Absurdities** (*e.g.*, nose missing in a picture)

Recall

Objectives:

1. Increase memory and attending skills

2. Provide means for him to discuss previous activities and events

3. Teach use of past tense

Procedure: Create a situation that highlights an action or activity and then ask Student what occurred. Initially, he will be asked immediately. Gradually, the delay between the action and the question will be increased.

At the start, it is helpful to have him describe what he is doing as he is performing the action. Also, time and place markers will facilitate recall.

Phase 1: **The teacher or Student should perform some action. Have him describe the action while it is underway.** Have him stop, wait a few moments then ask, "What did you do?" This will also teach past tense.

This can be prompted by first showing him a picture of the action he is about to do. When he has completed the action, have him select the correct picture in response to the question.

Phase 2: **Trips**. Send Student out of the room to do something. Initially the action should be significant, interesting and memorable. Have him return and ask him, "What did you do?"

Gradually lengthen the time between the event and the question, "What happened?" It may be necessary to provide prompts, such as, "What did we do in the **living room**?," "What did we do at the **mall**?," etc.

Phase 3: **Ask Student what occurred earlier in the day**. It will be necessary to find out what did occur so that he does not simply provide rote answers and so that you can verify what he says.

To prepare him for this, be sure to have him describe what he is doing at the time he does it. He should be asked what he did soon after and again from time to time to keep it in memory.

Here are some interesting places to go that will provide topics for recall and conversation:

> Stores/Malls
> Gymboree
> Discovery Zone
> Reading hour at the library
> Pet store
> Beach
> Park

Phase 4:   **Ask Student what occurred yesterday.** When the time is greatly lengthened, it may be helpful to prompt his response by showing him pictures including one depicting what occurred and have him select, "What did we do yesterday?"

Phase 5:   **Teach Student to ask others what happened in their day.**

Cross-Refer: Expressive Labeling-Actions
Expanding Language I
Conversation: Basic, Intermediate, Advanced

Quantitative Concepts

Objectives:

1. Develop academic skills

2. Increase quantitative reasoning skills

3. Provide means of solving quantitative problems in everyday life

4. Provide foundation for understanding money concepts

5. Expand expressive use of language concepts relating to quantity and measurement

A. **Stacking Rings and Nesting Cups**. SD: "Put on" or "put in." R: Student puts them together in the correct order.

B. **Arrange up to Five Objects by Size**: "Put these in order."

C. **Count 1-10 (left-to-right, one-to-one correspondence)**. SD: present objects and say "Count." R: Student touches each item and says number.

D. **Rote Counting 1-100**. SD: "Count to [10]." R: Student recites numbers in order. There are no objects present for this.

E. **Make it Equal (1-5) with Three-Dimensional Objects**. Present two cards to Student. One has a defined quantity of objects on it. Point to the other card (which has no objects on it) and tell him to make it equal.

F. **Match Quantities in Varying Configurations, with Varying Objects**. Use index cards with varying numbers of stickers on them. SD: "Put with [one]" *vs.* "Put with [three]. R: Student matches a card with one [red heart] to the card with one [yellow star] *vs.* matching a card with three [red hearts] to a card with three [yellow stars].

G. **Receptive Quantity (without counting) - Point to (1,2,3,4,5)**. Put out piles with varying numbers of objects. SD: "Point to [three]." R: Student points to the pile that has three objects.

1. Three-dimensional objects
2. Two-dimensional (pictures)

H.   **Expressive Quantity (without counting) - How many? (1,2,3,4,5)**. Put out a pile with 1-5 objects. Teacher points to the pile and asks, "How many?" Student answers with correct number without counting.
1.   Three-dimensional objects
2.   Two-dimensional objects

I.   **Symbols (numerals)**
1.   Receptive Identification: "Point to [three]"
2.   Expressive Labeling: "What number?"
3.   Matching Symbol to Quantity: "Put with same"
4.   Match number word to numeral and quantity: "Put with same."

J.   **Make it _____ (1-5)**. Put out a blank card and a tray with a large number of objects. Point to the blank card and say, "Make it [three]." Student should put [three] items on the card.

K.   **More vs. Less**. Put out two piles of objects. SD: "Point to more." R: Student points to the correct pile.
1.   With objects
  a.   <u>More</u>: 5 *vs.* 1
  b.   <u>More</u>: 4 *vs.* 1
  c.   <u>More</u>: 3 *vs.* 1
  d.   <u>Less</u>: 5 *vs.* 1
  e.   <u>Less</u>: 5 *vs.* 2
  f.   (1 or 2) *vs.* (3, 4, or 5) more and less
2.   With two-dimensional pictures
3.   Make it more/less
4.   Most/Least

L.   **Sequences: "Put these in order."**
1.   Puts consecutive number cards in order
2.   Puts nonconsecutive number cards in order
3.   What comes <u>Before/After</u> [number]? (with visual)
4.   What comes <u>Before/After</u> [number]? (no visual)

M.   **First/Last**
1.   Beginning and end of pictorial sequence
2.   Beginning and end of number or alphabet sequence
3.   Point to objects
4.   Carry out actions

N.   **Counts by 10, 2, and 5**. SD: "Count by [two's]. R: "[2, 4, 6, 8 . . .]"

O.   **Addition Facts**

P.   **Subtraction Facts**

Q.   **Adding *vs.* Subtracting**

R.   **Odd/Even**

S.   **Ordinal Numbers**

T.   **Story Problems**

Reading

Objectives:
1. Develop academic skills.
2. Increase means of communication.
3. Provide leisure activity.

Procedure: The teacher presents letters or words and has Student demonstrate understanding.

Prompts: Use position, verbal, pointing, or hand-over-hand prompts. Gradually fade prompts.

Entry criter: Student can match objects to objects, pictures to pictures, and pictures to objects. Ordinarily, he will have completed Receptive Labeling. However, a few students who get stuck on auditory associations can learn to make visual associations (*e.g.*, matching a word with an object).

Mastery crit: Student performs a response eight out of ten times correctly with no prompting. This should be repeated with at least one additional teacher.

Phase 1: Matching letters and numbers.

Phase 2: Matching word to word.

Phase 3: Matching single letters to word in left-to-right order.

Phase 4: Recite alphabet.

Phase 5: Receptive identification of uppercase letters.

Phase 6: Receptive identification of lowercase letters.

Phase 7: Expressive naming of uppercase letters.

Phase 8: Expressive naming of lowercase letters.

Phase 9: Put alphabet cards in order.

Phase 10:   **Saying sound letter makes.**   Teacher shows a card with a letter on it and asks, "What sound?"

Phase 11:   **Blending sounds.** Put out two or more letter cards, *e.g.,* **C - A - T**. Tell Student to read and point to each letter, one at a time. Student should say the sounds one by one as you move your finger. As you move your finger more quickly across the letters, he should blend the sounds together to make the word.

Phase 12:   **Matching word to item or picture.** You can make a game out of this by printing words on cards for items in the environment. Have Student read card and stick it on the appropriate item.

Phase 13:   **Receptive identification of words.**

Phase 14:   **Spelling words orally.**

Phase 15:   **Reading sentences.**

Phase 16:   **Matching phrases to pictures.**

Phase 17:   **Comprehension.** Have Student answer questions about what he reads.

           a)   Who [did action]?
           b)   What did [person] do?
           c)   Where?
           d)   How/Why?

Phase 18:   **Following written instructions.** Make up index cards with simple written instructions for tasks and activities that he commonly does around the house.

           a)   one-word instructions
           b)   two-word instructions
           c)   three-word instructions
           d)   complete sentences

Writing

Objectives:	1. Provide a means of communicating
	2. Develop academic skills
	3. Improve grapho-motor skills
Procedure:	Provide stimulus for student to make response on paper.
Prompts:	Use physical guidance, demonstration, verbal, pointing or position prompt. Gradually fade the prompts until Student can perform independently.
Entry criter:	Drawing, Reading
Mastery crit:	Student performs a response nine out of ten times correctly with no prompting. This should be repeated with at least one additional teacher.
Phase 1:	**Trace letters and numbers.** Use lined paper.
Phase 2:	**Traces, copies and writes name.** Start when Student can successfully perform Phase 1.
Phase 3:	**Copying letters and numbers.**
Phase 4:	**Writing letters and numbers.** Start when Student can successfully perform Phase 3 and Student can identify letters and numbers. The teacher tells Student, "Make [letter __]."
Phase 5:	**Matching single letters to word in left-to-right order.**
Phase 6:	**Copying from chalkboard at front of room.**
Phase 7:	**Taking dictation of words.**
Phase 8:	**Writing sentences in answer to questions.**
Cross-Refer:	Drawing Reading

Self-Help Skills

Objectives:

1. Increase independence in daily living skills

2. Develop age appropriate functioning

3. Facilitate social integration

Procedure:

First, it is important to follow a **task analysis**. All skills should be divided into teachable parts. This will simplify the skill and therefore reduce Student's frustration. It also ensures that he understands each individual step. More important, it helps promote consistency. It is **CRITICAL** that all teachers use the same steps in the same order as outlined in the task analysis.

A systematic and graduated teaching approach is also necessary for Student to fully learn and retain skills. Teaching complex skills all at once is not an effective teaching method.

Third, it is essential to follow the concept of **mastery**. That is, Student should be taught one step at a time. The next step should not be taught until the previous step has been mastered. A step is considered mastered once the step has been completed **independently (*i.e.*, no prompts of any kind are used)** for three consecutive sessions.

Fourth, when teaching, use the least intrusive prompt necessary. The prompt hierarchy that is typically used is the following:

> Gestural Prompt
> Indirect Verbal Prompt (*e.g.*, "keep going")
> Direct Verbal Prompt (*e.g.*, "get towel")
> Modeling
> Physical Guidance

Eventually the prompt should be faded, so that Student performs the task independently. Use differential reinforcement, giving greater reinforcement on steps that are performed with reduced assistance.

A final consideration is the timing of the teaching process. It is important that teaching be conducted under the most optimal conditions possible. That means teaching when Student and the teacher are likely to be most receptive and effective in their actions. It is important to teach at a time when he is not exhibiting problems and is interested and motivated to learn. Where possible, this should be at naturally occurring opportunities, but not at the expense of quality teaching. For example, getting ready for school is a naturally occurring moment for teaching dressing, but often is **NOT OPTIMAL** timing because of time pressure. Just before going outside to play is optimal, because you can take as long as you need and there is a built in natural reinforcer and natural reason for practicing the behavior.

Feeding/Eating
1. Drinks from cup with both hands, without assistance (B: 1-3)
2. Uses spoon to "scoop" food (B: 1-3)
3. Takes spoon from plate to mouth, with some spilling (B: 1-6)
4. Sucks from straw (B: 1-6)
5. Drinks from cup with one hand, without assistance (B: 1-6)
6. Uses fork (B: 2-0)
7. Uses spoon, without spilling (B: 2-0)
8. Uses side of fork for cutting soft foods (B: 3-0)
9. Holds fork in finger (B: 4-0)
10. Uses knife for spreading (B: 4-0)
11. Uses knife for cutting (B: 6-0)
12. Pouring

Undressing
1. Removes socks (B: 1-6)
2. Removes shoes (B: 1-6)
3. Removes coat (B: 2-0)
4. Removes shirt (B: 2-0)
5. Removes pants (B: 2-0)
6. Undresses, except for difficult "pull over" clothes (B: 3-0)
7. Removes sweater (B: 4-0)

Dressing
1. Puts on jacket (B: 2-6)
2. Puts on shoes (B: 2-6)
3. Puts on pants (B: 2-6)
4. Puts on socks (B: 3-0)
5. Puts on sweater (B: 3-0)
6. Dresses with little supervision (B: 3-0)
7. Dresses without supervision but needs help with fasteners (B: 4-0)
8. Dresses independently (B: 5-0)

Unfastening
1.   Unbuttons front buttons (B: 2-0)
2.   Unties bow (B: 2-0)
3.   Unsnaps front snaps (B: 3-0)
4.   Unzips (B: 3-0)

Fastening
1.   Buttons large front buttons (B: 3-0)
2.   Snaps front snaps (B: 3-0)
3.   Zips front zipper (B: 3-0)
4.   Attempts to lace shoes (B: 3-0)
5.   Buttons small front buttons (B: 3-0)
6.   Laces shoes (B: 4-0)
7.   Attempts to tie shoes (B: 4-0)
8.   Ties shoes (B: 5-0)

Bathing
1.   Dries hands, may need assistance (B: 2-0)
2.   Washes hands, may need assistance (B: 2-0)
3.   Dries hands, without assistance (B: 2-6)
4.   Dries face, may need assistance (B: 2-6)
5.   Washes hands, without assistance (B: 3-0)
6.   Washes face, with assistance (B: 3-0)
7.   Turns faucet on and off (B: 3-0)
8.   Adjusts water temperature, with assistance (B: 3-0)
9.   Dries face, without assistance (B: 3-0)
10. Washes face, without assistance (B: 4-0)
11. Bathes, with assistance (B: 4-0)
12. Dries self after bathing, without assistance (B: 4-0)
13. Bathes, without assistance (B: 6-0)

Grooming
1.   Attempts to brush teeth, with much assistance (B: 2-0)
2.   Brushes teeth, with assistance (B: 3-0)
3.   Brushes teeth, without assistance (B: 4-0)
4.   Brushes hair, with assistance (B: 4-0)
5.   Brushes hair, without assistance (B: 5-0)

Home Living
1.   Putting things away
2.   Simple food preparation (microwave, toaster, spreading, stirring, etc.)
3.   Chores (set table, take dishes to sink, take out trash, make/change bed, laundry, etc.)
4.   Cleaning table, window, wall
5.   Put dishes in sink, set table
6.   Caring for pets

Community

1. Pedestrian safety
2. Making purchases
3. Transportation
4. Correspondence
5. Safety/strangers/handling emergencies

Money Skills

1. Match coins
2. Receptive labels
3. Expressive labels
4. Making purchase

Using Telephone

Giving Messages

Get Requested Item And Deliver To Person

Grocery Shopping

Toilet Training

Entry criter: Student is able to sit for a prolonged period of time.

Procedure: Prior to training take Student off favorite liquids and reinforcers so as to increase their value during toilet training as well as consumption of liquids.

INDEPENDENT TOILETING (B: 2-6)

Phase 1:   1.   Place Student on the toilet and reinforce him with praise and fluids every two to three minutes for "good sitting." You can bring a variety of activities into the bathroom to keep him occupied. However, he should not be so occupied that he is unable to attend to body cues.

2.   Once Student voids, he should be praised profusely, given a highly preferred reinforcer and be allowed to leave the toilet to engage in a favorite activity for approximately ten minutes. However, he should remain in the bathroom during this time.

3.   A short time later (*e.g.*, ten minutes), he should return to the toilet to repeat the process again.

4.   If a long time passes with no voiding and he is getting uncomfortable, allow him to get up for a few minutes, but keep him in the bathroom. After a short time, have him return to sitting on toilet. It is **VERY** important to keep time off the toilet **BRIEF** and to monitor him **CLOSELY** during this time. You do **NOT** want an accident to occur during this time.

Progression Criterion: When Student appears to understand the relationship between toileting and reinforcement, move to the next phase.

Phase 2:   1.   Place him in a chair next to the toilet with no underwear or pants.

2.   Reinforce him with praise and fluids every two to three minutes for "good sitting."

3.   Wait for him to get up on his own to go to toilet.

DO NOT PROMPT EVEN IF HE/SHE EXHIBITS A
TREMENDOUS NEED TO VOID!!!   OTHERWISE HE/SHE
WILL LIKELY BECOME PROMPT DEPENDENT.

4.   When he voids in the toilet, the following should occur:
   a.   He should be praised profusely (*i.e.*, a circus should come to town!!!).
   b.   He can leave the bathroom for a short time (*e.g.*, ten minutes) to engage in a favorite activity.
   c.   The chair should be gradually moved further away from the toilet.
   d.   One article of clothing should be added (*e.g.*, first time=underpants; next time=pants; etc.).

5.   If an accident happens, the following should occur:
   a.   If you see an accident starting to happen, resist the temptation to rush him to the toilet, otherwise he will become dependent!!!
   b.   He should clean body parts, wet clothing and the environment where the accident took place.
   c.   He should review the correct use of the toilet, approximately five times.
   d.   The chair should be moved to the previous placement.
   e.   One article of clothing should be removed.

**Progression
Criterion:**   When Student is fully dressed and away from the bathroom move to the next phase.

Phase 3:   1.   Check Student every 30 minutes to see if he has dry and clean pants. Praise him profusely for dry and clean pants.

2.   If an accident occurs, use the procedure described in Phase 2 above.

3.   When he voids in the toilet, reinforce him heavily (see above).

4.   The time between "dry pants checks" should be lengthened (*e.g.*, 60 minutes, two hours, four hours, six hours, etc.).

Habit Training

1.   Identify Student's toileting schedule.

2.   Take him to the bathroom 15 minutes prior to typical toileting time.

3.   Place Student on the toilet without clothing and reinforce him with praise and fluids every two to three minutes for "good sitting."

4.   Once he voids, he should be praised profusely and allowed to leave the toilet to engage in a favorite activity.

5.   If he does not void within 30 minutes, then have him return to the previous activity.

6.   Return Student to toilet every hour until voiding occurs.

7.   If an accident occurs outside the toilet training session, the following should occur:
    a.   He should clean body parts, wet clothing and the environment where the accident took place.
    b.   He should review the correct use of the toilet, approximately five times.

Shaping Independent Toileting (for a child already habit trained)

1.   This phase would be used if previous attempts at toilet training have resulted in Student being dependent on prompts or a schedule to get him to use the toilet. However, he should be able to remain dry between toilet visits and void immediately when placed on the toilet.

2.   The training can start 30 to 60 minutes after he has last voided. (This decreases the delay between the start of the session and the first occasion to use the toilet.) It helps to have given him extra fluids in advance. Start by bringing him into the bathroom and placing him on a chair near the toilet. Reinforce him with praise and fluids every two to three minutes for appropriate behavior. While he is sitting on the chair, you can play, sing, look at books, do drills, watch videos, etc. However, allow frequent lulls in the activity, so as not to inhibit any initiation.

3.   Wait for him to get up on his own to go to toilet. It is very tempting to prompt him to go to the toilet, but the goal here is to eliminate prompt dependence so the best policy is **DO NOT PROMPT**. If it seems unavoidable that you must give him a prompt, make the prompt nonverbal, such as a gesture, and fade it as quickly as possible.

4.   When Student voids in the toilet, he should be praised profusely (*i.e.*, a circus should come to town!!!). He can then leave the area for a while (*e.g.*, 10-30 minutes.).

5.   With each new success, the chair should be gradually moved further away from the toilet before Student is brought back to the bathroom.

6.   If an accident occurs during toilet training or outside the session, the following should occur:
    a.   He should clean body parts, wet clothing and the environment where the accident took place.
    b.   He should review the correct use of the toilet, approximately five times (*i.e.*, practice getting up from his chair and sitting briefly on the toilet).
    c.   The chair should be moved to the previous placement.

Nighttime Toilet Training

1.   Purchase training pad (moisture sensing mattress pad with alarm), available from Night Trainer (800) 544-4240 or Mattell Toy (905) 501-5149.

2.   Determine if the bell will wake him. If not, it will be necessary to connect the pad to a louder bell.

3.   When bell activates, make sure he is fully awake and assist him in voiding as needed.

4.   Have him assist in the cleaning pad before going back to sleep.

Bowel Movement Difficulties

Withholding

1.   Reduce possible power struggles (*e.g.*, anger, demands, etc.).

2.   Identify reinforcers Student will earn when he "chooses" to void.

3.   Identify large reinforcers he will earn when he is independently toilet trained.

4.   Place reinforcers in prominent spot so Student can view reinforcers.

5.   Ask him once daily how he earns the reinforcers.

6.   If an accident occurs, the following should occur:
    a.   He should clean body parts, wet clothing and the environment where the accident took place.
    b.   He should review the correct use of the toilet, approximately five times.

Diaper Rituals

1.   Provide Student diaper to use in the bathroom.

2.   Once he is voiding in the diaper while in the bathroom, start having him sit on the toilet (still with diaper on) until he has a bowel movement.

3.   After he voids in the diaper, have him place contents in the toilet.

4.   Cut opening in the diaper until he is no longer wearing diapers.

School Checklist

Items to be rated on daily report:

_____ Follows classroom rules

_____ Keeps hands to self

_____ Keeps eyes on teacher at appropriate times

_____ Follows individual directions

_____ Follows group and conditional directions

_____ Follows routine without direction or model (*e.g.*, puts backpack away)

_____ Stays around other children; does not isolate

_____ Responds to conversation of other children

_____ Initiates play

_____ Initiates verbal interaction

_____ Not going too fast with activity

_____ Remains patient when has to wait

_____ Remains in designated place at work time; stays in line (queue)

_____ Clarity of language

_____ Notices what other children do and takes cue from them

_____ Recites in unison

_____ Shares toys

_____ Asserts self when another child tries to take something away

_____   Refrains from stereotyped behavior (stim)

_____   Plays appropriately with toys

_____   Stays on task for work

_____   Stays with assigned (or chosen) play activity

Appendices

CURRICULUM ASSESSMENT

Name: _____

OBSERVATION 1   Date: _____   Evaluator: _____

Comments: _____

_____

OBSERVATION 2   Date: _____   Evaluator: _____

Comments: _____

_____

OBSERVATION 3   Date: _____   Evaluator: _____

Comments: _____

_____

OBSERVATION 4   Date: _____   Evaluator: _____

Comments: _____

_____

SKILL CODES:

M: <u>Mastery level</u>
   M1: Not Ready
   M2: Learning
   M3: Mastered
    G: Generalized

N: Number of items mastered

H: Highest level accomplished

I: Itemized list of items mastered

C: Complexity (e.g., number of
   blocks in design)

BEHAVIOR CODES:

%: Percent of occurrence

S: <u>Severity</u>
   S1: Severe
   S2: Moderate
   S3: Mild

F: <u>Frequency</u>
   HR: Hourly
   DY: Daily
   WK: Weekly
   MO: Monthly

D: Average Duration

Appendix A

BEHAVIOR		OBS 1	OBS 2	OBS 3	OBS 4
Tantrums	F	HR = 4/total			
	S	S2			
Self-Abuse	F	—			
	S	—			
Aggression	F	—			
	S	—			
Self-stim	F	HR			
	S	S3			
Other Major Disruptive Behavior (Specify):	F	HR —			
turning out lights in classroom	S	S3			
Other Major Disruptive Behavior (Specify):	F	—			
	S	—			
Leaves Work Area/chair	F	HR			
	S	S2			
Hands and Feet Restless	F	HR			
	S	S2			
Attention Span (Average Duration)	D	5 min.			
Eye-to-Face-Contact: looking on request	%	15%			
looking when name is called	%	50%			
looking when talking or listening	%	20%			
Looking at Task Materials	%	50%			
Follows Simple Directives with Gestures	%	50%			
Compliance: come here from 5 feet away	%	50%			
come from across room	%	30%			
come from other parts of house	%	—			
come when outside at close distance in confined area	%	—			
come outside at longer distance	%	—			
sit down	%	25%			
stand up	%	25%			
hands down	%	15%			

BEHAVIOR (cont.)		OBS 1	OBS 2	OBS 3	OBS 4
Retrieve Objects (May Be with Gesture; No Distractor):					
from table	M	m2			
from floor next to table	M	m2			
from 5 feet away	M	m2			
from across room	M	m1			
Waiting:					
To hear instruction	M	m2			
While teacher gets reinforcer	M	m2			
While adult completes necessary activity	M	m2			
To take turn in highly preferred activity	M	m2			
Stays on Task for Independent Work (Specify Task & Duration):					
task 1: Social Story	D	5-10min			
task 2: Reading	D	15 min			
task 3: Math	D	0 min			
Performs Skills in Different Situations:					
varied language and materials	M	M1			
different people	M	m2			
different places	M	M2			
increase distance between therapist and child;	M	m2			
Generalize Compliance and Appropriate Behavior (e.g., at supermarket, park, friends' and relatives' homes)	M	——			

ATTENTION TRACKING		OBS 1	OBS 2	OBS 3	OBS 4
Shell Game [teacher hides object under cup & student finds it: 1) one distractor; 2) two; 3)three or more	H				

		OBS 1	OBS 2	OBS 3	OBS 4
NONVERBAL IMITATION	M				
Object Manipulation	N				
Large Motor Movements	N				
Out of Chair	N				
Small Motor	N				
Continuous Chain	M				
Finer Discriminations	N				
Two-step Chains	M				
Crossing Over	N				
Two Responses at Once	N				
Three-step Chains	M				
Imitates action in video: ____Single discrete action; ____2 step (simultaneous); ____3 step; ____Continuous chain; ____2step delayed; ____3step delayed;					
Freeze frame video	N				
Action in photo	N				
Imitates another person	N				

		OBS 1	OBS 2	OBS 3	OBS 4
BLOCK IMITATION	M				
Building a Tower	C				
Discriminates Colored Shapes	M				
Sequential Steps	C				
Pre-built Structure	C				
1" Cubes	C				
Uniform blocks	C				
Copying 2-d Design	C				
Creating Specific Structures	N				
	C				
Design from Memory	C				

GROSS MOTOR (specify task):		OBS 1	OBS 2	OBS 3	OBS 4
Task 1:	M				
Task 2:	M				
Task 3:	M				
Task 4:	M				
Task 5:	M				

FINE MOTOR (specify task):		OBS 1	OBS 2	OBS 3	OBS 4
Task 1:	M				
Task 2:	M				
Task 3:	M				
Task 4:	M				
Task 5:	M				

		OBS 1	OBS 2	OBS 3	OBS 4
MATCHING	M	—			
Object-to-Object	N	—			
Picture-to-Picture (identical objects)	N	8			
Picture-to-Picture (identical actions)	N	8			
Color	M	M2			
Form (circle, square, triangle)	M	—			
Size (big vs. little)	M	—			
Object-to-Picture (identical)	N	—			
Picture-to-Object (identical)	N	—			
Find same (pointing)	M	M2			
Multiple dimensions (identical color/shape/size combinations)	M	—			
Sorting: starter provided for each pile	C	—			
no starter provided	C	—			
Non-identical objects (3-D)	N	—			
Non-identical pictures (2-D)	N	—			
Non-identical object-to-picture and picture-to-object	N	—			
Non-identical actions	N	—			
Quantity	N	—			
Associations	N	—			
Emotions	N	—			
Prepositions	N	—			
Letters, Numbers, Words	M	M2			

		OBS 1	OBS 2	OBS 3	OBS 4
DRAWING	M				
Control of Pen	M				
Continuous Circles vs. Up/Down Strokes	M				
Fill Within Outline	C				
Painting	C				
Trace Lines, Circles	M				
Connect Dots	M				
Copy Lines, Circles	M				
Use Ruler	M				
Copy Drawings of Familiar Objects	N				
Draw Shapes Free Hand	N				
Draw Familiar Objects Freehand	N				

		OBS 1	OBS 2	OBS 3	OBS 4
PLAY					
Interaction games (peek-a-boo, pat-a-cake)	M				
Cause and Effect Toys (Jack-in-box)	M				
Completion/Developmental Toys (ring stack)	M				
Puzzles	C				
Trucks/Cars/Trains	I				
Construction Toys: (blocks, Legos, tinker toys, etc.)	I				
Play Sets (e.g., farm)	I				
Turn Taking Games (Barnyard Bingo, Don't Break the Ice)	I				
Movement Games (duck-duck-goose, tag)	I				
Songs, dance (London Bridge, Ring-a-Rosie, etc.)	I				
Ball Play: 1) Roll; 2) Throw; 3) Catch; 4) Kick	I				
Books	M				
Board Games	I				
Imaginary Play (Doctor, Power Rangers)	I				

		OBS 1	OBS 2	OBS 3	OBS 4
RECEPTIVE INSTRUCTIONS	M				
Instructions with Contextual Cue	N				
Follows Pictorial Directions: ____1 Step; ____2 Step; ____3 Step; ____Extended Sequence	N				
Object Manipulation	N				
In Chair	N				
Pretend Actions	N				
Out of Chair, Same Room	N				
Go to Other Room and Return	N				
Go to Other Room, Perform Action & Return	N				
Say vs. Do	M				
Two-step Instructions	M				
Three-step Instructions	M				
Conditional directions	N				

		OBS 1	OBS 2	OBS 3	OBS 4
RECEPTIVE LABELS	M				
Requests	M				
Body Parts	N				
Objects	N				
Pictures of Objects	N				
Pictures of Action	N				
Pictures of People	N		✓		
People (3-D)	N				
Retrieves Two Items	M				
Color	N				
Shape	N				
Size	M				
Combined Color/Object Discrimination	M				
Two Attributes Combined	M				
Three Attributes Combined	M				
Pictures of Places (home & community)	N				
Emotions (see Emotions section)	M				

		OBS 1	OBS 2	OBS 3	OBS 4
INITIATING INTERACTION/COMMUNICATION:	M				
Choices/Functional Communication:					
chooses from items displayed (takes item)	M				
points to desired item from those offered	M				
selects icon and delivers to adult (staged)	M				
selects icon and delivers to adult (incidental)	M				
discriminates between icons	C				
states desires - item present	M				
states choice - item not present	M				
Communication Temptations:					
Staged	N				
Incidental	M				
Asking Questions:					
What is it?	N				
Who is it?	N				
Where is it?	N				
What are you doing?	N				
What's in there?	N				
Where are you going?	N				
Who has it?	N				

		OBS 1	OBS 2	OBS 3	OBS 4
VERBAL IMITATION	M				
Spontaneous Babbling	M				
Oral Motor Imitation	N				
Object Manipulation with Sound	N				
Temporal Discrimination	M				
Match Sounds	N				
Blends	N				
Sounds Without Visual Cue	M				
Imitates Modulation:					
volume	M				
duration	M				
pitch	M				
inflections	C				
Chains	N				
Words with Difficult Sounds	N				
Imitation of Two Word Phrases	N				
Imitation of 3-5 Word Sentences	M				

		OBS 1	OBS 2	OBS 3	OBS 4
EXPRESSIVE LABELS	M				
Requests	N				
Body Parts	N				
Objects	N				
Pictures of Objects	N				
Pictures of Action	N				
In Vivo Action	N				
Pictures of People	N				
People (3-D)	N				
Color	N				
Shape	N				
Size	N				
Pictures of Places around Home	N				
Pictures of Locations around Community	N				
Emotions (see Emotions section)	M				

✳

		OBS 1	OBS 2	OBS 3	OBS 4
BASIC CONVERSATIONAL SKILLS	M	—			
Responds to Greeting: 1) looks; 2) says hi; ③) says hi + name	H	3			
Manding	N	—			
Sentence stems:					
I want...	M	m ⅃			
It's a ...	M	m⅃			
That's a ...	M	m⅃			
I see ...	M	m⅃			
I have ...	M	m⅃			
Commenting (look at this, I did it, etc.)	N	○			
Acknowledges statement (oh, what?, etc.)	N	○			

		OBS 1	OBS 2	OBS 3	OBS 4
ASSERTIVENESS	M				
Desires (see Communication Tempt.)	M				
Expresses displeasure	M				
Acts to prevent unwanted action of others	M				
Conviction: 1) objects; 2) actions; 3) attributes	I				
Identifies and Corrects Teacher Mistake	M				
Resists Inappropriate Suggestion	N				

		OBS 1	OBS 2	OBS 3	OBS 4
YES/NO	M				
Desires ("Do you want cookie?")	M				
Negation: Don't do this	M				
Don't [action]	M				
Say vs. Don't say	M				
Not (touch not apple)	M				
Objects ("Is this a truck?")	M				
Persons ("Is this Daddy?")	M				
Actions ("Is mommy standing?")	M				
Attributes ("Is this red?")	M				
Concepts ("Is this the corner?")	M				
Answers True/false (or Yes/no) Questions about Things That Are Not Visible	M				
Answers Questions That Are Partially True	M				

		OBS 1	OBS 2	OBS 3	OBS 4
JOINT ATTENTION	M				

		OBS 1	OBS 2	OBS 3	OBS 4
EMOTIONS	M				
Non-identical Matching	N				
Recognizing Emotion Portrayed in Pictures	N				
Labels Emotion in Pictures	N				
Demonstrating Specific Emotions	N				
Labels Emotions Portrayed by Others	N				
Stating How He Feels	N				
Identifying Causes for Emotions	M				
Carry out Action to Create Emotion in Another Person	M				
Labels Emotions and Causes in Self and Others in Incidental Situations	M				
Identifies Appropriate Response to Emotional Situation	N				

		OBS 1	OBS 2	OBS 3	OBS 4
PRAGMATIC GESTURES	M				

		OBS 1	OBS 2	OBS 3	OBS 4
ATTRIBUTES	M				
Physical Properties	I				
Gender	M				
Loud/Soft	M				
Spatial Concepts	I				
Quantitative Concepts	I				
Other Opposites	I				
Logical Connectors (and, or)	M				

	M	OBS 1	OBS 2	OBS 3	OBS 4
FUNCTIONS	M				
Student Shows Action for 3-d Object	N				
What Do You [Action] with? Points to Object	N				
What Is a [Object] for? (Object Visible/verbal Response)	N				
What Do You [Action] with? Points to Picture	N				
Student Shows Action for 2-d Item	N				
What Do You [Action] with? (Verbal Response)	N				
What Is a [Object] for? (Object Not Visible/verbal Response)	N				
What Do You [Body Function] with?	N				
What Do You Do with Your [Body Part]?	N				
What Do You Do in [Room]?	N				
Where Do You [Action]?	N				

	M	OBS 1	OBS 2	OBS 3	OBS 4
CATEGORIES	M				
Matching/sorting	N				
Receptive (Point to Animal)	N				
Expressive (What Group Is Dog)	N				
Name Something That Is [Category]	N				

	M	OBS 1	OBS 2	OBS 3	OBS 4
GENERAL KNOWLEDGE AND REASONING I	M				
Associations - Matching Two Related Objects (3-D)	N				
Associations - Matching Two Related Items (2-D)	N				
Auditory Discrimination - Matches Item to Live Sound: Chooses from objects	N				
Chooses from pictures	N				
Gives answer with no visual	N				
Auditory Discrimination - Matches Item to Recorded Sound: Chooses from objects	N				
Chooses from pictures	N				
Gives answer with no visual	N				
Associates Action with person/animal/character: What does animal say?	N				
What does character eat?	N				
What does character do?	N				
What/Who says [sound]?	N				
Who eats [item]?	N				
Who [does action]?	N				

GENERAL KNOWLEDGE AND REASONING I (cont.)		OBS 1	OBS 2	OBS 3	OBS 4
Locations:					
Receptive room identification (own home) 2-D	N				
Expressive labels for rooms in own home 2-D	N				
Goes to named room	N				
Names room where he is	N				
Receptive identification of generic rooms (2-D and 3-D)	N				
Expressive labeling of generic rooms (2-D and 3-D)	N				
Receptive identification of community locations (2-D and 3-D)	N				
Expressive labeling of community locations (2-D and 3-D)	N				
Community Helpers:					
Receptive identification of person	N				
Expressive labeling of person	N				
What does a [person] do?	N				
Who [does role]? ___points to picture ___verbal response	N				
Where would you see [person]? ___points to picture ___verbal response	N				
What does a [person] use? ___points to picture ___verbal response	N				
Opposites (verbal SD only, no visual):					
Puts together (2-D)	N				
What is the opposite of: Points to opposite	N				
What is the opposite of: Names (no visual)	N				
Composition:					
Sorts items made of same material	N				
What is made of [material]: Points	N				
What is [object] made of?	N				
Names something made of [material]	N				
Describes Person (person present)	C				
	N				
Identifies Person Who Has Characteristic(s)	C				
	N				
Describes Animal/Object (object visible)	C				
	N				
Identifies Animal/Object Who Has Characteristic(s)	C				
	N				

		OBS 1	OBS 2	OBS 3	OBS 4
GENERAL KNOWLEDGE AND REASONING II	M				
Describes Person or Object (item not in view)	N				
Identifies Person or Object Who Has Characteristic(s) (item not in view)	N				
Associations:					
Verbal question-verbal response (What goes with shoe?)	N				
Explains Why Two Items Go Together	N				
Why/when Do We Do Action?	N				
What Do You Do When?	N				
Where Do We Go to...	N				
Impossible Tasks	N				
Absurdities:					
Identifying	M				
Explaining	M				
Correcting	M				
Identifies Item Missing in Picture	N				
Riddles	M				
Analogies	M				
Patterning - Adds next Item to a Series: 1) ABAB; 2) AABB; 3) ABBABB; 4) AABAAB; 5)ABCABC	I				
Coding	C				

		OBS 1	OBS 2	OBS 3	OBS 4
SAME/DIFFERENT	M				
Give Me Same vs. Give Me Different	M				
Find Same or Different vs. Comparison Object	M				
Tells Whether Two Items Are Same or Different	M				
Answers Why Same or Different	M				
Answers Why Same or Different for Items That Are Both Same and Different	M				

		OBS 1	OBS 2	OBS 3	OBS 4
PREPOSITIONS	M				
Receptive:					
On top: 1) objects; 2) self; 3) pictures	M				
Under: 1) objects; 2) self; 3) pictures	M				
Inside: 1) objects; 2) self; 3) pictures	M				
Beside/next to: 1) objects; 2) self; 3) pictures	M				
Between: 1) objects; 2) self; 3) pictures	M				
Behind: 1) objects; 2) self; 3) pictures	M				
In front: 1) objects; 2) self; 3) pictures	M				
Expressive:					
On top: 1) objects; 2) self; 3) pictures	M				
Under: 1) objects; 2) self; 3) pictures	M				
Inside: 1) objects; 2) self; 3) pictures	M				
Beside/next to: 1) objects; 2) self; 3) pictures	M				
Between: 1) objects; 2) self; 3) pictures	M				
Behind: 1) objects; 2) self; 3) pictures	M				
In front: 1) objects; 2) self; 3) pictures	M				

		OBS 1	OBS 2	OBS 3	OBS 4
PRONOUNS	M				
Receptive:					
My vs. Your	M				
His/her: 1) persons; 2) pictures	M				
Their/our/your	M				
Me/you ("Point to me/you")	M				
Him/her ("Give [object] to him/her"; "Point to him/her)	M				
Expressive:					
My vs. Your	M				
His/hers	M				
Theirs/ours	M				
I/you	M				
He/she	M				
They/we	M				
Nominative/Possessive combinations ("You are touching my nose")	M				

		OBS 1	OBS 2	OBS 3	OBS 4
EXPANDING LANGUAGE	M				
It's a [Object]	M				
I Have [Object]	M				
I See [Object]	M				
I See [Object] and [Object]	M				
I See [Multiple Objects Around Room, Etc.]	M				
I See [Multiple Items in Complex Picture]	M				
Verb/object Combinations	N				
Noun/verb Combinations	N				
Pronoun/verb	N				
Adjective/object	N				
Adjective/adjective/object	N				
Noun/verb/object	N				
Pronoun/verb/object	N				
It's a [Adjective/object]	M				
I See [Adjective/object]	M				
I Have [Adjective/object]	M				
It's a [Adjective/adjective/object]	M				
I See [Adjective/adjective/object]	M				
I Have [Adjective/adjective/object]	M				
Adjective/object/preposition/object	M				
Subject/verb/object/descriptor	M				
Verb Tenses: Present	M				
Past	M				
Future	M				
Plurals: Receptive nouns	M				
Expressive nouns	M				
Expressive verbs	M				
Uses singular and plural nouns and verbs in sentences	M				

		OBS 1	OBS 2	OBS 3	OBS 4
"I DON'T KNOW"	M				
Answers I Don't Know to Unknown Question: What is it?	M				
Who is it?	M				
Where is it?	M				
Seeks information in response to question: What is it?	M				
Who is it?	M				
Where is it?	M				
Answers I Don't Know to Incidental Questions	M				
I Don't Understand	M				

		OBS 1	OBS 2	OBS 3	OBS 4
INTERMEDIATE CONVERSATIONAL SKILLS	M				
Answers Open-Ended Rote Questions (What's your name?)	N				
Answers Subjective Questions (What's your favorite...?)	N				
Answers Yes/No Questions (Are you a boy?)	N				
Answers Simple Conversational Questions (What did you do last night?)	N				
Answers Multiple Choice Questions	N				
Asks Reciprocal Questions	N				
Statement/Statement	N				
Statement/Question	N				
Statement/Negative Statement	N				
Statement/Statement/Question	N				

		OBS 1	OBS 2	OBS 3	OBS 4
ASKING QUESTIONS	M				
What is it?	M				
Who is it?	M				
Where is it?	M				
What are you doing?	M				
What's in there?	M				
Where are you going?	M				
Who has it?	M				

		OBS 1	OBS 2	OBS 3	OBS 4
SEQUENCING	M				
Three Card Sequence	N				
Ordering Three Alphabet Cards	M				
Ordering Three Number Cards	M				
Four Card Sequence	N				
What Happens Next?	M				
Five and Six Card Picture Sequence	M				
Ordering 4-6 Alphabet Cards	M				
Ordering 4-6 Number Cards	M				

		OBS 1	OBS 2	OBS 3	OBS 4
TEMPORAL CONCEPTS	M				
First/Last:					
Beginning and end of pictorial, number, or alphabet sequence	M				
Beginning and end of line of characters/people	M				
What did you touch first vs. last	M				
What did you do first vs. last	M				
Beginning and end of number or alphabet sequence	M				
Before/After:					
What comes before vs. after number	M				
What comes before vs. after letter	M				
What comes before vs. after day	M				
What comes before vs. after picture in sequence	M				
What did you do before vs. after middle action	M				
Carries out instruction with before vs. after	M				

IMAGINATION & STORY TELLING	M	OBS 1	OBS 2	OBS 3	OBS 4
Makes Animal Sound	N				
Acting like an Animal	N				
Child Pretends to Do Something	N				
Child Identifies Action That Therapist Portrays	N				
Acting out Roles: Librarian, Winchell's Clerk, Bus Driver, Etc.	I				
What Could this Be? (Creative Use of Ordinary Objects.)	N				
Drawing Pictures	I				
Making Structures and Objects with Legos/blocks	I				
Sequence Narration - "Tell Me the Story": 1) one scene; 2) two scenes; 3) three scenes; 4) four-six scenes	H				
Tell a Story with Picture Prompts	I				
Complete a Story/sequence - "What's Going to Happen?"	M				
Taking Turns Adding to Story	M				
Create a Story	M				

CAUSE & EFFECT	M	OBS 1	OBS 2	OBS 3	OBS 4
Answers Why Question for Live Demonstration	N				
Missing Sequence	M				
What Happened Prior to the Sequence	M				
What Is Likely to Happen next	M				
Inference about Action Portrayed in Picture	M				
Answers Why Question from General Knowledge and Information (intraverbal)	M				

		OBS 1	OBS 2	OBS 3	OBS 4
COMPREHENSION	M				
Observing:					
What (3-D and 2-D)	M				
What Color (3-D and 2-D)	M				
What vs. What Color	M				
Who (3-D and 2-D)	M				
Who vs. What	M				
What Doing (3-D and 2-D)	M				
Who vs. What vs. What Doing	M				
Where (3-D and 2-D)	M				
Who vs. What vs. What Doing vs. Where	M				
Which (3-D and 2-D)	M				
Who vs. What vs. What Doing vs. Where vs. Which	M				
How (3-D and 2-D)	M				
Who vs. What vs. What Doing vs. Where vs. Which vs. How	M				
Listening and Reading:					
Who vs. What doing	M				
Who vs. What doing vs. What vs. What Color	M				
Where (3-D and 2-D)	M				
Who vs. What Doing vs. What vs. What Color vs. Where	M				
Who vs. What Doing vs. What vs. What Color vs. Where vs. When	M				
Who vs. What Doing vs. What vs. What Color vs. Where vs. When vs. Which	M				
Who vs. What Doing vs. What vs. What Color vs. Where vs. When vs. Which vs. Why	M				
Who vs. What Doing vs. What vs. What Color vs. Where vs. When vs. Which vs. Why vs. How	M				

		OBS 1	OBS 2	OBS 3	OBS 4
ADVANCED CONVERSATIONAL SKILLS	M				
Tell vs. Ask	M				
Non-verbal Conversational Behavior	M				
Verbal Manners	M				
Lists Items for Topics	M				
Responding to Simple Questions	M				
Reciprocates Statements	M				
Asks Questions	M				
Interjects Information	M				
Identifying Interests	M				
Initiates Conversation	M				
When Peers Become Disinterested	M				

		OBS 1	OBS 2	OBS 3	OBS 4
SOCIAL AWARENESS	M				
Learning from Modeling Prompt: Verbal	M				
Visual	M				
Greetings: Responds	M				
Initiates	M				
Sharing and Cooperation: Taking turns	M				
Losing graciously	M				
Identify Which Person in Group: Holds a particular object	M				
Has certain attribute (hair color, blue sweater, etc.)	M				
Is performing a particular action	M				
Said a particular phrase	M				
Other information (e.g. likes, dislikes)	M				
Attends to Verbal Input in Group Setting: Remains in designated place during group activity	D				
Performs action in unison with group	%				
Sings song in unison with group	%				
Looks toward speaker	%				
Responds to group questions	%				
Follows group directions	%				
Giving Information to Group/circle Games	M				
Seeks Information by Asking a Question	M				

		OBS 1	OBS 2	OBS 3	OBS 4
OBSERVATIONAL LEARNING	M				
Modeling as Prompt	M				
Awareness: Identifies person holding object	M				
Identifies person with physical characteristic	M				
Identifies person doing action	M				
Identifies person who made statement	M				
Listens to Trials Given to Another Person (can answer question about what has happened): What did [person] do?	M				
Who [does action]?	M				
What does [person] like to do?	M				
Listens to Incidental Information	M				
Observes Events in Environment (can answer question about what has happened)	M				
Detects Incorrect Information	M				
Which One Did Person See?	M				
Group Instructions: Everyone	M				
Conditional	M				
I Do/Not Me	M				
Information Acquisition-Verbal	M				
Drawing Inference-Verbal	M				
Information Acquisition-Visual	M				
Drawing Inference-Visual	M				
Describes Peers Interests	M				

		OBS 1	OBS 2	OBS 3	OBS 4
SOCIALIZATION SKILLS	M				

		OBS 1	OBS 2	OBS 3	OBS 4
MEMORY	M				
Visual Memory (Delayed Matching)	M				
Giving Multiple Objects (Receptive Labels)	M				
What's Missing?	M				
Remembers Three Objects after 10 Sec. Exposure	M				
Recall	M				
Remembers Words to Song	M				
Recount a Familiar Story (E.g. Three Little Pigs)	M				

Appendix A

QUANTITATIVE CONCEPTS		OBS 1	OBS 2	OBS 3	OBS 4
Stacking Rings and Nesting Cups	M				
Arrange up to Five Objects by Size	M				
Count 1-10 (Left-to-right, One-to-one Correspondence)	H				
Rote Counts To: _____	H				
Make it Equal with Three Dimensional Objects	M				
Match Quantity:					
Identical configuration	H				
Non-Identical configuration	H				
Receptive Quantity:					
3-D Objects	H				
2-D objects	H				
Expressive Quantity:					
3-D objects	H				
2-D objects	H				
Symbols (numerals):					
Receptive Identification	H				
Expressive Labeling	H				
Matching Symbol to Quantity	H				
Match number word to numeral and quantity	H				
Make it [quantity]/Give Me [quantity]	H				
More vs. Less:					
Receptive discrimination	M				
Make it more/less	M				
Most vs. least	M				
Sequences:					
consecutive numbers	H				
nonconsecutive numbers	M				
What comes Before/After [number]	M				
Counts By: ____10; ____2; ____5	I				
Addition Facts	H				
Subtraction Facts	H				
Adding vs. Subtracting	M				
Odd/even	M				
Ordinal Numbers	H				
Story Problems	M				

		OBS 1	OBS 2	OBS 3	OBS 4
TIME CONCEPTS	M				
Calendar: Days of the week	M				
Months	M				
Year	M				
Today/tomorrow/yesterday	M				
Weekend/weekday	M				
Next week/last week	M				
When do you _____ ?: morning; afternoon; evening; night;	M				
Seasons	M				
Holidays	M				
Telling Time: 1) To the hour; 2) To the half-hour; 3) To the quarter-hour; 4) To nearest 5 minutes	H				

X **READING**

		OBS 1	OBS 2	OBS 3	OBS 4
Matching:					
Letters	M	m 2			
Word to word	M	m 2			
Single letters to word in left-to-right order	M	m 2			
Recite Alphabet	M	m 3			
Receptive Identification:					
Uppercase letters	N	—			
Lowercase letters	N	—			
Expressive Naming:					
Uppercase letters	N	—			
Lowercase Letters	N	—			
Puts Alphabet Cards in Order	C	—			
Saying Sound Letter Makes	N	8			
Blending Sounds	M	m 2			
Matching Word to Picture/Objects	M	m 2			
Receptive Identification of Words	N	—			
Spelling Words Orally	N	—			
Reading Sentences	M	m 1			
Matching Phrases to Pictures	M	m 1			
Comprehension:					
Who [did action]?	M	m 2			
What [did person Do]?	M	m 1			
Where?	M	m 2			
How/Why?	M	m 0			
Following Written Instructions:					
One word commands	N	—			
Two word commands	N	—			
Three word commands	N	—			

WRITING		OBS 1	OBS 2	OBS 3	OBS 4
Trace letters and numbers on lined paper	M				
Traces, copies and writes name	M				
Copying letters and numbers	M				
Writing letters and numbers	M				
Matching single letters to word in left-to-right order.	M				
Copying from chalkboard at front of room.	M				
Taking dictation of words.	M				
Writing sentences in answer to questions.	M				

SELF-HELP SKILLS		OBS 1	OBS 2	OBS 3	OBS 4
Eating:					
Spoon/fork	M				
Drinking from cup	M				
Pouring	M				
Drink from straw	M				
Spread/cut with knife	M				
Dressing:					
Clothes off	M				
Clothes on	M				
Unfastening (snap; button; zip)	M				
Fastening	M				
Shoes off	M				
Shoes on	M				
Tie shoes	M				
Toileting:					
Habit Trained	M				
Initiates Toileting	M				
Dry at Night	M				
Hygiene:					
Washing face/hands	M				
Brushing teeth	M				
Grooming hair	M				
Bathing	M				
Home living:					
Putting things away	I				
Simple food prep (microwave, toaster, spreading, stirring, etc.)	I				
Chores (set table, take dishes to sink, take out trash, make/change bed, laundry, etc.)	I				
Cleaning table, window, wall	I				
Put dishes in sink, set table	I				
Care for pets	M				
Community:					
Pedestrian safety	M				
Making purchases	M				
Transportation	M				
Correspondence	M				
Safety/strangers/handling emergencies	M				

SELF-HELP SKILLS (cont.)		OBS 1	OBS 2	OBS 3	OBS 4
Money Skills:					
Match coins	M				
Receptive labels (1¢, 5¢, 10¢, 25¢, 50¢, $1, $5, $10, $20)	N				
Expressive labels	N				
Making purchase	M				
Using Telephone	M				
Giving Messages	M				
Get Requested Item and Deliver to Person	M				
Grocery Shopping	M				

DAILY DATA SUMMARY

PROGRAM: _____

PHASE: _____

DISCRETE TRIAL DATA

PROGRAM: _____   PHASE: _____

(+) CORRECT   (–) INCORRECT   (P) PROMPT   (0) NO RESPONSE   (OT) OFFTASK

Appendix C

OVERVIEW OF PROGRAMS

Date:

PERFORMANCE EVALUATION

Staff: _____   Date: ___/___/___

Evaluator: _____   Child: _____

Reason for Evaluation: _____

1 = Rarely Occurred/   2 = Partially met/   3 = Usually Occurred/
    Definite concerns   Needs improvement   Adequate/Acceptable

(Items marked with * cannot usually be rated from a single direct observation.)

BEHAVIOR SHAPING

		1	2	3
1.	Provides positive reinforcement at times to strengthen and maintain appropriate task behavior.			
2.	Does not use threats or bribes.			
*3.	Uses proactive teaching to promote appropriate alternative behavior.			
4.	Corrects disruptive behavior as needed.			

SITUATION

		1	2	3
1.	Teaching materials were ready and organized			
2.	Setup of physical environment and level of distractions were appropriate for student			
3.	Teaching location was varied and natural settings were used (as appropriate for student)			

TASK

		1	2	3
1.	Tasks were appropriate to student's functioning level			
2.	Tasks were broken down into component parts			
*3.	The teacher understands the purpose of the program			

Appendix E

INSTRUCTIONS (SD)	1	2	3
1. Instructions were appropriate to child's functioning (e.g., level of complexity, explicitness, etc.)			
2. Natural tone of voice was used			
3. Words used corresponded to desired response			
4. Variation/consistency in instruction corresponded to child's level of functioning			
5. Appropriate time was given for response (e.g., **approximately** 3-5 seconds)			

FEEDBACK/CONSEQUENCE	1	2	3
1. Feedback was as immediate as needed by student			
2. Consequences were effective			
3. Student's responses were correctly evaluated			
4. The frequency of reinforcement was optimal (often enough to be effective, but faded as quickly as possible)			
5. Differential consequences were utilized (for quality of response, attention, decreased prompt, etc.)			
6. Informational feedback was used			
7. If tangible reinforcers were used, they were accompanied by social reinforcers in order to effectively develop social reinforcement value			
8. Contingencies were consistently implemented			
9. Used varied reinforcers			

INTERTRIAL INTERVAL	1	2	3
1. Each trial was separate			
2. The intertrial interval was optimal (good pacing; student allowed sufficient time to be reinforced)			

PROMPT		1	2	3
1.	Timing of prompts was optimal (normally this means accompanying or immediately following the instruction)			
2.	Just enough assistance was given to ensure success, but never more than needed			
3.	If the first prompt did not work, more intrusive prompts were provided			
4.	Prompts were used to avoid prolonged failure by providing necessary assistance			
5.	Prompted trials were followed by non-prompted or reduced-prompted trials			
6.	The appropriate type of prompt was used (e.g., demonstration, verbal model, physical guidance, within-stimulus, etc.)			
7.	When the student made an error due to inattention or off-task behavior, prompts were only used when the behavior could not be corrected with consequences			
*8.	There were systematic attempts to fade prompts			
9.	Was sensitive to inadvertent prompts (e.g., positional, glances, patterns, mouthing answers, etc.)			

ESTABLISHING ATTENTION		1	2	3
1.	Reinforced good attention when it occurred			
2.	Timed onset of trials optimally to shape better attending			
*3.	Followed plan to promote independent direction of attention			

MAXIMIZING PROGRESS:
(MADE LEARNING FUN AND NATURAL)

		1	2	3
1.	Session length was appropriate; timing and duration of breaks was appropriate			
2.	Arranged task order so that difficult tasks occurred between easier tasks			
3.	Ended session on a pattern of successes			
4.	Created behavioral momentum			
5.	Incorporated a good balance of play into the overall program			
6.	Made therapy as natural as possible (e.g., models natural language)			
7.	Attempted to facilitate generalization as quickly as possible			
8.	Adjusted training based upon student's behaviors and performance			
9.	Approach was enthusiastic			
10.	Used interesting and preferred materials			
11.	Did not bore the student by continuing a program that was already mastered			
12.	Rewarded student for good attending and performance by ending drills sooner			
13.	Interspersed tasks as appropriate			

ADDITIONAL COMMENTS (as needed)

_____

_____

_____

_____

_____

_____

Appendix E

As appropriate, comment on these general work habits as demonstrated in overall work performances with multiple clients:

PROFESSIONAL GROWTH	1	2	3
1. Is an eager and active learner			
2. Makes valuable contributions at clinics			
3. Seeks growth			

RELATIONSHIPS	1	2	3
1. Works well as member of clinical team			
2. Is responsive to feedback			
3. Relationships with parents are within appropriate boundaries			

RESPONSIBILITY & PROFESSIONAL BEHAVIOR	1	2	3
1. Is punctual			
2. Regular attendance is good			
3. Notifies family as appropriate for cancellations			
4. Uses time wisely			
5. Dresses professionally			

ADDITIONAL COMMENTS (as needed)

_____

_____

_____

_____

_____

_____

_____

_____

_____

_____

_____

_____

_____

_____

_____

_____

_____

_____

_____

Staff Acknowledgement: _____   Date: ___/___/

Appendix E

PROGRAM DESCRIPTION

PROGRAM: _____   INTRODUCED: _____   MASTERED: _____

General Procedure: _____

_____

_____

_____

_____

_____

Start	Teacher says/does:	Student says/does:
	Sd 1)	R 1)
	Sd 2)	R 2)
	Sd 3)	R 3)
	Sd 4)	R 4)
	Sd 5)	R 5)

Prompts: _____

_____

_____

_____

Comments: _____

_____

_____

_____

TRACKING FORM

PROGRAM: _____   PHASE: _____

Item	Response	Started	Mastered	Comments
1				
2				
3				
4				
5				
6				
7				
8				
9				
10				
11				
12				
13				
14				
15				
16				
17				
18				
19				
20				

Appendix G